Haematology
Lecture Notes

Haematology
Lecture Notes

Deborah Hay

DPhil, MRCP, FRCPath
Nuffield Department of Clinical Laboratory Science
Radcliffe Department of Medicine
University of Oxford
Oxford, UK

Andrew King

DPhil, MRCP, FRCPath
Department of Haematology
Cambridge University Hospitals NHS Foundation Trust
Cambridge, UK

Michael Desborough

DPhil, MRCP, FRCPath
Department of Haematology
Oxford University Hospitals NHS Foundation Trust
Oxford, UK

Radcliffe Department of Medicine
University of Oxford
Oxford, UK

Eleventh Edition

WILEY Blackwell

This eleventh edition first published 2023
© 2023 John Wiley & Sons Ltd

Edition History
John Wiley & Sons Ltd (10e, 2018; 9e, 2013)

Registered Offices
John Wiley & Sons, Inc., 111 River Street, Hoboken, NJ 07030, USA
John Wiley & Sons Ltd, The Atrium, Southern Gate, Chichester, West Sussex, PO19 8SQ, UK

Editorial Office
The Atrium, Southern Gate, Chichester, West Sussex, PO19 8SQ, UK

For details of our global editorial offices, customer services, and more information about Wiley products visit us at www.wiley.com.

Wiley also publishes its books in a variety of electronic formats and by print-on-demand. Some content that appears in standard print versions of this book may not be available in other formats.

Library of Congress Cataloging-in-Publication Data
Names: Hay, Deborah, 1977- author. | King, Andrew, (MRCP, FRCPath, DPhil), author. | Desborough, Michael, author.
Title: Lecture notes. Haematology / Deborah Hay, Andrew King, Michael Desborough.
Other titles: Haematology
Description: Eleventh edition. | Hoboken, NJ : Wiley, 2023. | Preceded by Lecture notes. Haematology / Christian Hatton, Deborah Hay, David M. Keeling. Tenth edition. 2017. | Includes bibliographical references and index.
Identifiers: LCCN 2022032874 (print) | LCCN 2022032875 (ebook) | ISBN 9781119841203 (paperback) | ISBN 9781119841210 (adobe pdf) | ISBN 9781119841227 (epub)
Subjects: MESH: Hematologic Diseases | Blood Physiological Phenomena
Classification: LCC RC636 (print) | LCC RC636 (ebook) | NLM WH 120 | DDC 616.1/5–dc23/eng/20220826
LC record available at https://lccn.loc.gov/2022032874
LC ebook record available at https://lccn.loc.gov/2022032875

Cover Design: Wiley
Cover Image: © ImageFlow/Shutterstock

Set in 8.5/11pt UtopiaStd by Straive, Chennai, India

Printed in Singapore
M118964_290822

Contents

Preface to the 11th edition

Since the last edition of *Haematology Lecture Notes*, the practice of clinical and laboratory haematology has continued to evolve rapidly. This is reflected in some significant updates for this new edition, led by two new authors with an interest in medical education. As well as a new focus on changes to the blood count in non-haematological disease, there is an updated section on innovative cellular therapies for haematological malignancies (including CAR T therapies) and expanded chapters on haemostasis and anticoagulation.

This content is complemented by new online interactive clinical cases which apply and test the key principles discussed in each chapter. These take the form of case-based multiple choice questions, with over 150 questions available.

As always, we are grateful to the previous authors and to our colleagues for figures and advice, and to our students for their helpful comments on the text.

About the companion website

This book is accompanied by a companion website:

www.wiley.com/go/Hay/Haematology/11e

This website includes:

- Interactive case study multiple-choice questions
- Suggestions for further reading.

1

An introduction to haematopoiesis

LEARNING OBJECTIVES

After reading this chapter, you should be able to:

- ✔ describe the site and process of formation of blood cells
- ✔ understand the concept of a stem cell, and the idea of lineage specification of blood cells
- ✔ recognize the different types and functions of mature blood cells
- ✔ describe the basic structure of lymph nodes
- ✔ define B cells and T cells through their respective receptor gene rearrangements
- ✔ understand that malignant diseases of haematological cells derive from their recognizable normal counterparts.

An introduction to the blood and its diseases

An appreciation of blood and its normal components is essential for the care of patients in nearly every clinical specialty. Simple tests of haematological function inform our understanding of the responses to infection and inflammation, nutrition and gastrointestinal dysfunction, as well as renal and liver disease, and can sometimes provide the earliest indicators of malignant disease in tissues which are otherwise clinically hard to assess. This alone makes an understanding of basic haematology essential for every doctor.

Beyond this, haematology also encompasses some of the most common acquired and inherited disorders responsible for morbidity and mortality around the world, and some of the most aggressive and yet treatable malignancies. It has also provided transformational insights into the molecular basis of disease that have informed therapeutics in many specialties.

This opening chapter provides an overview of the formation and function of the cellular components of blood, which will be needed for each of the subsequent sections of this text.

The formation of blood

As the developing embryo grows, it starts to require a means of delivering oxygen to tissues for respiration. The circulation and blood develop at the same time, from around 3 weeks' gestation, and there are close links between the cellular origins of the first blood cells and the vasculature.

Haematology Lecture Notes, Eleventh Edition. Deborah Hay, Andrew King and Michael Desborough.
© 2023 John Wiley & Sons Ltd. Published 2023 by John Wiley & Sons Ltd.
Companion website: www.wiley.com/go/Hay/Haematology/11e

Haematopoietic stem cells originate in the para-aortic mesoderm of the embryo. Primitive red blood cells, platelet precursors and macrophages are initially formed in the vasculature of the extraembryonic yolk sac, before the principal site of haematopoiesis shifts to the fetal liver at around 5–8 weeks' gestation. The liver remains the main source of blood in the fetus until shortly before birth, although the bone marrow starts to develop haematopoietic activity from as early as 10 weeks' gestation.

After birth, the marrow is the sole site of haematopoiesis in healthy individuals. During the first few years of life, nearly all the marrow cavities contain red haematopoietic marrow, but this recedes so that by adulthood, haematopoiesis is limited to marrow in the vertebrae, pelvis, sternum and the proximal ends of the femora and humeri, with minor contributions from the skull bones, ribs and scapulae (Figure 1.1). It is the posterior superior iliac spine of the pelvis – a bony landmark readily palpable in most individuals - which is the usual site of bone marrow biopsy for the clinical assessment of the process of haematopoiesis.

Although the sites of haematopoiesis in the adult are therefore relatively limited, other sites retain their capacity to produce blood cells if needed. In conditions in which there is an increased haematopoietic drive (such as chronic haemolytic anaemias and chronic myeloproliferative disorders), haematopoietic tissue will expand and may extend into marrow cavities that do not normally support haematopoiesis in the adult. Foci of haematopoietic tissue may also appear in the adult liver and spleen and other tissues (known as extramedullary haematopoiesis).

Haematopoietic stem cells

The process of haematopoiesis needs to generate adequate numbers of specialised blood cells throughout life from a small pool of precursor cells. This is accomplished using the unique properties of haematopoietic stem cells.

Long-term haematopoietic stem cells (HSCs) in the bone marrow are capable of both self-renewal and differentiation into the progenitors of individual blood cell lineages. The progenitor cells of individual lineages then undergo many rounds of division and further differentiation in order to yield populations of mature blood cells. This process can be represented as a hierarchy of cells, with HSCs giving rise to populations of precursor cells, which in turn give rise

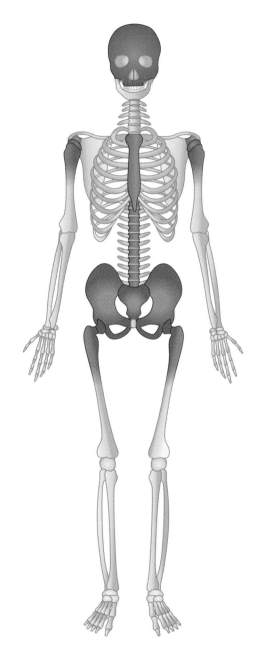

Figure 1.1 The red shading indicates the position of red (blood-forming) marrow in the adult. The posterior superior iliac spine of the pelvis is the usual site of bone marrow biopsy for clinical assessment of the process of haematopoiesis.

to cells increasingly committed to producing a single type of mature blood cell (Figure 1.2). Thus, the immediate progeny of HSCs are the multipotent progenitor cells, which have limited self-renewal

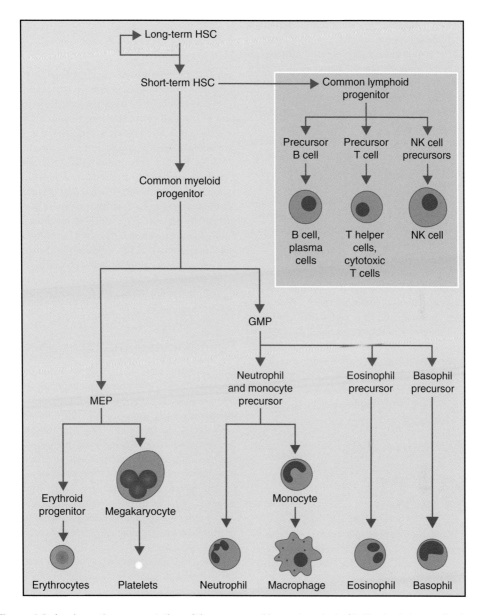

Figure 1.2 A schematic representation of the process of haematopoiesis. Multipotent stem cells give rise to lymphoid (pink) and myeloid (blue) lineages. The myeloid lineage further divides into granulocytic, erythroid and megakaryocytic (platelet) lineages. As cells progress through this process of differentiation, they accrue more functional specialization and lose their multipotency. GMP, granulocyte macrophage progenitor; HSC, haematopoietic stem cell; MEP, megakaryocyte/erythroid progenitor; NK, natural killer.

capacity but retain the ability to differentiate into all blood cell lineages. Although there is still debate about exactly how lineage-restricted subsequent precursors are, the concept of sequential and irreversible differentiation is widely accepted. In Figure 1.2, the HSC is seen giving rise to two major lineages: the lymphoid lineage, in which a common lymphoid progenitor gives rise to B cells, T cells and natural killer (NK) cells; and a myeloid lineage, with a common myeloid progenitor giving rise to red cells, granulocytes and platelets. The division of haematopoiesis into myeloid and lymphoid compartments is fundamental to an understanding of haematological disease.

The process of haematopoiesis outlined above has several advantages. First, it permits the massive expansion of cell numbers needed to maintain an adequate population of mature blood cells. It also means that the production of each type of mature blood cell can be controlled individually, tailoring production to specific physiological requirements. Finally, it requires relatively little proliferative activity on the part of the long-term HSCs themselves, thereby minimizing the risk of developing mutations in these crucial cells during DNA replication and cell division.

Haematopoietic stem cells were first detected and defined functionally through experiments in which a subset of cells from the bone marrow was shown to produce blood cells of all lineages when transplanted into lethally irradiated mice, which have no haematopoietic potential of their own. Subsequent work has used cell surface markers and flow cytometric techniques (see Chapter 7) to define this population: positivity for the cell surface marker CD34 combined with negativity for CD38 describes a population of multipotential cells that is capable of regenerating all cell lineages from the bone marrow. The cell surface marker CD34 is also used to isolate cells with multipotency and self-renewal capacity for autologous and allogeneic stem cell transplantation (see Chapter 12).

Differentiating blood cells

Precisely how the ultimate lineage choice of differentiating progenitor cells is determined remains a subject of research. It has been argued that factors intrinsic to the HSC itself, such as stochastic fluctuations in transcription factor levels, may direct lineage specification. However, it is also known that proper regulation of HSCs and progenitor cells requires their interaction with extrinsic factors, such as non-haematopoietic cells in the bone marrow niche (e.g. endothelial cells and osteoblastic progenitors). HSCs and progenitor cells are not randomly distributed in the marrow, but exist in ordered proximity relative to mesenchymal cells, endothelial cells and the vasculature. Signalling from these non-haematopoietic cells, plus physicochemical cues such as hypoxia and blood flow, are therefore likely to influence the transcriptional activity and fate of HSCs. It is clear, however, that the process of lineage specification is accompanied by a gradual reduction in the multipotency of the cell.

Myelopoiesis

Signalling through myeloid growth factors such as granulocyte-macrophage colony stimulating factor (GM-CSF) is essential for the survival and proliferation of myeloid cells. The specification of the myeloid lineage is also known to require the interaction of a series of specific transcription factors, including C/EBPα, RUNX1-core binding factor complex and c-Myb. As well as being essential for the normal formation of myeloid cells, it is becoming clear that an appreciation of these factors and others like them is critical for an understanding of myeloid diseases such as acute myeloid leukaemia (see Chapter 8).

The separation of the erythroid and megakaryocytic components of myelopoiesis requires the action of transcription factors GATA1, NF-E2 and SCL, and signalling through the growth factors thrombopoietin and erythropoietin.

Granulocytes and their function

Granulocytes, cells of the innate immune system characterized by the presence of specific cytoplasmic granules containing microbicidal and immunologically active molecules, are the most abundant white cells in the blood. The maturation of the normal bone marrow is outlined in Figure 1.3, with the least mature granulocytic cell, the myeloblast, passing through a series of successive stages termed promyelocytes (Figure 1.3b), myelocytes (Figure 1.3c), metamyelocytes and band forms. Cell division occurs in myeloblasts, promyelocytes and myelocytes, but not normally in metamyelocytes or band cells.

As well as a reduction in the size of the cell and the development of granules containing agents essential for their microbicidal function, the maturing granulocyte also gradually begins to adopt its characteristic nuclear segmented shape (Figure 1.4).

Mature neutrophils have the ability to migrate to areas of inflammation (chemotaxis), where they become marginated in the vessel lumen and pass into the tissues through interaction with selectins, integrins and other cell adhesion molecules. Once primed by cytokines such as tumour necrosis factor α (TNFα) and γ-interferon (IFNγ), neutrophils are able to phagocytose opsonized microbes, and destroy them by deploying their toxic intracellular contents. This release of reactive oxygen species (the 'respiratory burst') provides a substrate for the enzyme myeloperoxidase (MPO), which then generates

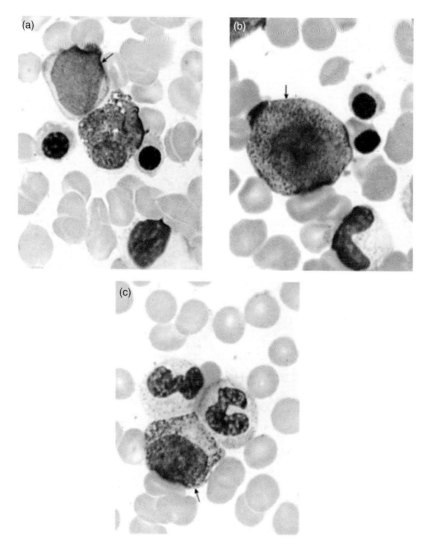

Figure 1.3 Neutrophil precursors from normal bone marrow. (a) Myeloblast (arrowed); the other nucleated cells near the myeloblast are an eosinophil (centre) and two polychromatic erythroblasts. (b) Promyelocyte (arrowed); the other nucleated cells are two polychromatic erythroblasts and a metamyelocyte. (c) Myelocyte (arrowed); there are two neutrophil band cells adjacent to the myelocyte. May-Grünwald-Giemsa (MGG) staining is used throughout for blood films.

hypochlorous acid with direct cytotoxic effects. The granules of neutrophils also contain an array of anti-microbial agents, including defensins, chymotrypsin and gelatinases.

Eosinophils, a subset of granulocytes with bright pink granules on haematoxylin and eosin-stained (H&E) blood films, have a similar ability to phagocy-tose and destroy micro-organisms, but are classically associated with the immune response to parasitic infection. They are often found in high numbers in patients with allergy and atopy. Interleukin 5 (IL-5)

signalling appears to be critical for their differentia-tion from granulocyte precursors.

Basophils are the least common of the granulo-cytes. They contain very prominent cytoplasmic granules which have stores of histamine and heparin as well as proteolytic enzymes. They are involved in a variety of immune and inflammatory responses, but it is unusual to see a marked elevation or depression in their numbers in reactive conditions. Figure 1.5 shows examples of each of the normal mature granulocytes.

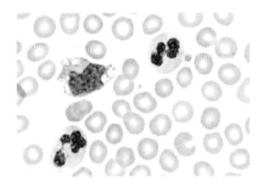

Figure 1.4 Monocyte and two neutrophil granulocytes – the monocyte has a pale, greyish-blue vacuolated cytoplasm.

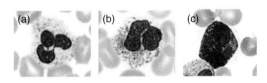

Figure 1.5 Mature granulocytes. (a) Neutrophil: note the polylobed nucleus and fine cytoplasmic granules. (b) Eosinophil, with a typical bilobed nucleus and pinkish orange (eosinophilic) granules. (c) Basophil, with granules so darkly staining as to obscure the nuclear contours

Monocytopoiesis and monocyte function

Functionally, monocytes have a variety of immune roles. As the precursors of tissue macrophages and dendritic cells, their roles include phagocytosis, antibody presentation to other immune cells and contributing to the cytokine milieu. Phagocytosis of micro-organisms and cells coated with antibody (with their exposed Fc fragments) and complement occurs via binding to Fc and C3b receptors on the surface of monocytes and macrophages. Bacteria and fungi that are not antibody-coated are phagocytosed after binding to mannose receptors on the phagocyte surface. As with neutrophils, the killing of phagocytosed micro-organisms by monocytes/macrophages may involve superoxide dependent and O_2-independent mechanisms.

The cell classes belonging to the monocyte–macrophage lineage are, in increasing order of maturity, monoblasts, promonocytes and monocytes (with the latter only typically seen in the blood), and tissue macrophages. Their synthesis is controlled in part by the activity of GM-CSF.

Megakaryocytes and platelet function

Megakaryocytes are the cells that give rise to platelets, the cellular fragments needed for primary haemostasis. During megakaryocyte formation, driven by the action of the growth factor thrombopoietin (TPO), there is replication of DNA without cell division. This leads to the generation of very large cells that are markedly polyploid, with a lobulated nucleus. A mature megakaryocyte is illustrated in Figure 1.6. Large numbers of platelets are formed from the cytoplasm of each mature megakaryocyte; these are rapidly discharged directly into the marrow sinusoids. The residual 'bare' megakaryocyte nucleus is then phagocytosed by macrophages.

TPO is the key regulator of normal platelet production. This protein, which is produced by the liver, binds to TPO receptors on the megakaryocyte membrane. Downstream signalling through mechanisms including the JAK/STAT pathway allows an increase in megakaryocyte ploidy, and also cytoplasmic maturation such that increased numbers of platelets are released. TPO is also able to bind to the surface of platelets themselves; thus, when platelet numbers are high, TPO is sequestered on the platelet membranes,

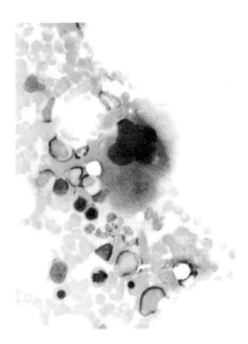

Figure 1.6 Mature megakaryocyte (centre). This is a very large cell with a single lobulated nucleus. Compare the size of the megakaryocyte with that of the other nucleated marrow cells in this figure.

leaving less available to act on the megakaryocytes to promote further platelet production. In this way, a negative feedback loop is created, maintaining platelet numbers within stable limits.

The fundamental role of platelets is in primary haemostasis, through their interactions with von Willebrand factor and the exposed collagen of damaged endothelial surfaces (see Chapter 13).

Erythropoiesis and red cell function

The specification of the erythroid lineage requires a balanced interaction between transcription factors GATA1 and other haematopoietic transcription factors, including PU.1 and FOG1. Once committed to an erythroid fate, the expansion of erythroid precursors takes place, driven largely by signalling through the erythropoietin receptor.

The hormone erythropoietin (epo) is expressed principally in the cortical interstitial cells of the kidney, where its transcription is modulated in response to hypoxaemia. The transcription factor hypoxia inducible factor (HIF-1) is induced in cells exposed to hypoxaemic conditions and enhances expression of the erythropoietin gene. Increased levels of erythropoietin are therefore available to interact with the epo receptor on red cell progenitor membranes, activating an erythroid-specific signal transduction cascade and leading to enhanced proliferation and terminal differentiation of erythroid cells.

Morphologically, the differentiation and maturation of erythroid cells are shown in Figure 1.7. Proerythroblasts are early erythroid progenitors in the bone marrow recognizable by their large size, their dark blue cytoplasm, their dispersed nuclear chromatin and nucleoli. As the cells mature, they become smaller with less basophilic cytoplasm (Figure 1.7).

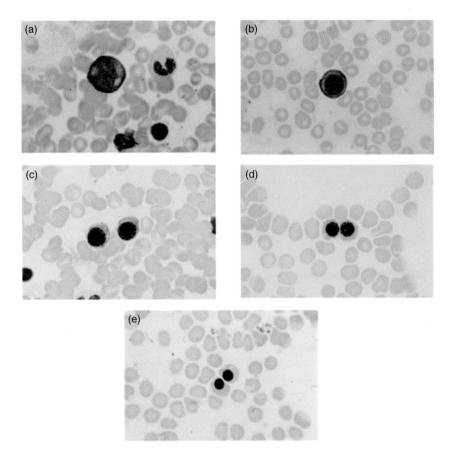

Figure 1.7 (a) Proerythroblast, (b) basophilic normoblast, (c) two early polychromatic normoblasts, (d) two late polychromatic normoblasts and (e) two very mature late polychromatic normoblasts. The condensed chromatin in the basophilic normoblast is slightly coarser than in the proerythroblast. The nuclei of the late polychromatic normoblasts contain large masses of condensed chromatin.

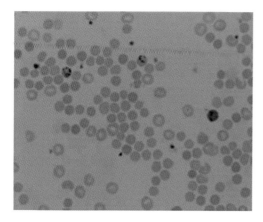

Figure 1.8 Reticulocytes in peripheral blood stained supravitally with brilliant cresyl blue. Note the reticulum of precipitated ribosomes.

Cell division continues until the cells reach the late polychromatic normoblast stage, when cells extrude their nucleus. At this point, the cell is termed a reticulocyte (Figure 1.8) and is released from the marrow into the peripheral blood. Reticulocytes are characterized by their slightly larger size and bluish staining (due to higher RNA content) contrasted with mature red cells. After 1–2 days in circulation, reticulocytes lose their remaining ribosomes and become mature red cells.

The red cell function is to carry oxygen, bound to the haem moiety of haemoglobin, from the lungs to the peripheral tissues. The details of haemoglobin structure and function (and diseases resulting from perturbation of these) are discussed further in Chapter 3.

Lymphopoiesis

B cells are needed for antibody production, and T cells for cell-mediated immunity. They are thought to arise from multilymphoid progenitor cells in the fetal marrow. Although incompletely characterized, these progenitors are known to feature CD45 and CD7 cell surface markers. The transcription factor Ikaros has been shown to be critical for lymphopoiesis in mouse models; Pax5 is among several transcription factors needed for B-cell development, while GATA3 and Notch signalling are essential for T-cell maturation.

B-cell development

The development of B lymphocytes commences in the fetal liver and fetal marrow. Here, progenitor B cells develop into pre-B cells (defined by the presence of the cytoplasmic μ chain of the B-cell receptor, see below) and then into mature B cells. During this time, the genes for the immunoglobulin light and heavy chains are rearranged, allowing the production of immunoglobulins with a wide array of antigenic specificities. Subsequent B-cell maturation requires antigen exposure in the lymph nodes and other secondary lymphoid tissues, with the mature B cell having the capacity to recognize non-self-antigens and produce large quantities of specific immunoglobulin.

Immunoglobulin structure and gene rearrangement

The defining feature of B-cell development is the production of immunoglobulin with a wide range of antibody specificities. Immunoglobulins are made up of two identical heavy chains and two identical light chains (either κ or λ) (Figure 1.9). The five major classes of immunoglobulin – IgA, IgG, IgM, IgD and IgE – are defined by their heavy chains (α, γ, μ, δ and ε) and the two heavy chains and two light chains are held together in a Y-shaped structure. The amino terminal portions of the heavy and light chains are known as 'variable' regions (V_H or V_L), because differences in their amino acid sequence create unique antigen-binding sites, each of which can recognize a different epitope. In contrast, the carboxy terminal regions are the 'constant' regions (CH or CL), because their structure is similar for all immunoglobulins of the same class. The enzyme papain cleaves the immunoglobulin molecule into an Fc fragment consisting of the carboxy terminal regions of the heavy chain and two Fab fragments containing the antigen-binding site. A number of cell types (e.g. splenic macrophages) possess Fc receptors that can bind the Fc portion of immunoglobulin molecules.

Human plasma contains all types of immunoglobulin, but IgG is present at the highest concentration. IgA is the second most common type of immunoglobulin and is found at mucosal surfaces in the gut and respiratory system. IgM represents <10% of the immunoglobulin found in plasma and is the antibody most commonly produced during a primary immune response. IgM has a very large molecular weight

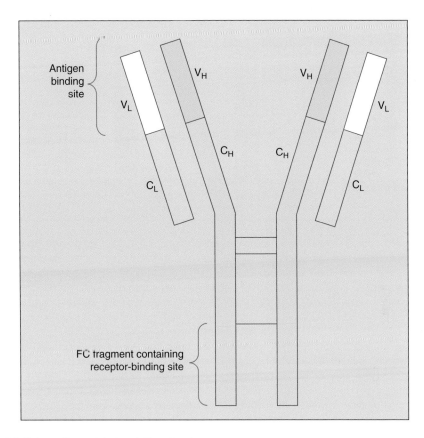

Antigen binding site

V_L

V_H

V_H

V_L

C_H

C_H

C_L

C_L

FC fragment containing receptor-binding site

Figure 1.9 Schematic model of an IgG molecule.

(approximately 900 000 kDa) and is pentameric in structure – relevant in the clinical presentation of Waldenström macroglobulinaemia (see Chapter 9).

Antibody diversity

Immunoglobulin gene rearrangement is the mechanism by which a single variable gene (V_H or V_L) in either a heavy or light chain gene complex is juxtaposed to genes encoding the constant region (C_H or C_L), generating differences from one immunoglobulin molecule to another in antigen-binding specificities (Figure 1.10). Diversity is increased by the introduction of randomly generated sequences, as well as by mutations within the variable regions. In consequence, a B-cell clone can synthesize immunoglobulin molecules with unique antigen-binding sites. It may be added that at different stages of differentiation, a single B cell can synthesize heavy chains with different constant regions but with the same

variable regions and thus antigen specificity. Thus, a B cell can start by expressing IgM but following antigen binding can produce IgG, IgA or IgE.

B-cell selection and maturation

B cells arising from progenitor cells in the bone marrow make their way to the germinal centre of lymphoid tissue, where they encounter antigen already bound to dendritic cells. If the surface immunoglobulin (sIg) on the B cells binds this antigen, the cross-linking provides a survival signal. Otherwise, the B cells undergo apoptosis, a process that ensures selection of 'useful' B cells, which become memory B cells and plasma cells.

Lymph node structure

Lymph nodes contain densely packed T and B lymphocytes, organized in a manner that allows the

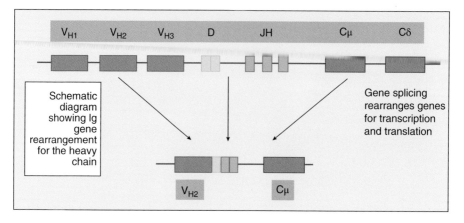

Figure 1.10 A diagram illustrating gene rearrangement enabling antigen-binding diversity. During differentiation, a single B cell can synthesize heavy chains with different constant regions coupled to the same variable region. Note that it is the genetic locus itself that undergoes rearrangement, not merely the transcripts it generates. The T-cell receptor (TCR) undergoes gene rearrangement in a very similar way in T cells. C, constant region gene; D, diversity gene; JH, joining sequence; VH, variable gene.

presentation of antigen to produce an effective immune response. In addition to having a blood supply, lymph nodes receive 'afferent' lymphatic vessels, which drain antigen-rich lymph from the tissues.

Within the unstimulated lymph node, resting B cells are organized into structures called primary follicles (Figure 1.11). When exposed to antigen (e.g. from micro-organisms), these structures enlarge and germinal centres develop, comprising proliferating B cells lying within a meshwork of follicular dendritic cells. Surrounding the follicles are sheets of lymphocytes, which become increasingly rich in T cells towards the lymph node medulla. The medulla contains several types of lymphocytes, including plasma cells.

Other lymphoid tissue

Lymphoid tissue is found in many sites other than lymph nodes. These sites include tissues directly exposed to external pathogens (e.g. respiratory and gastrointestinal tracts) and also central sites such as the bone marrow and spleen. The spleen is the largest single lymphoid mass in the body, and its white pulp component bears relation to a lymph node, though with no afferent lymphatic; instead, the lymphoid cells in the white pulp of the spleen respond to antigen borne directly in the blood, making it critical in the early immune response to

bacteraemia. The red pulp of the spleen is the site of removal of senescent red cell and platelets from the circulation.

Plasma cells are found in many lymphoid tissues, particularly at sites where they can secrete immunoglobulin into the circulation or mucous secretions (e.g. into the respiratory or gastrointestinal tracts). The spleen is the principal source of antibodies in the circulation.

T-cell development

T cells originate from lymphoid precursors in the marrow and fetal liver. These earliest immature T cells express neither CD4 nor CD8 and undergo rearrangement of the T-cell receptor genes to permit cell surface expression of the TCR. As with the surface immunoglobulin or B-cell receptor, the process of rearrangement yields a vast collection of potential TCRs, with the ability to recognize a wide range of different antigens. The TCR is formed from two polypeptide chains, usually α and β or less commonly γ and δ. Interaction of the TCR and a binding ligand results in T-cell activation and proliferation.

During the process of maturation, T cells migrate from the bone marrow to the thymus, acquire both CD4 and CD8 cell surface markers (termed 'double-positive' thymocytes) and undergo a process of positive selection to ensure the survival only of those

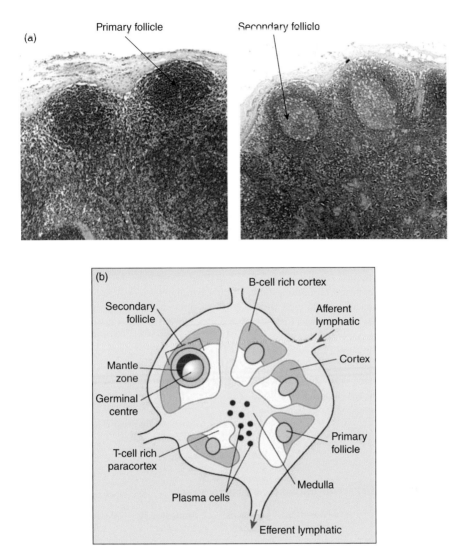

Figure 1.11 (a) Histological section through a lymph node and (b) illustration of a stylized lymph node.

that are able to interact adequately with major histocompatibility complex (MHC) molecules on antigen-presenting cells. T cells that interact with MHC class I become CD8 positive only, while those that interact with MHC class II downregulate their CD8 expression and become CD4 T cells. Any T cells that fail to recognize MHC will die by apoptosis, and the same fate awaits cells that bind with very high affinity. As a consequence, the T cells that emerge from the thymus all carry TCRs with an intermediate affinity for 'self' MHC molecules. This ensures

that they will subsequently continuously bind to (and disengage from) self-MHC molecules. However, if alteration of the MHC molecule by the presence of a peptide (e.g. from a virus) increases the affinity of TCR binding, the cell presenting the peptide with the MHC molecule will become the target for specific recognition and killing.

CD4+ lymphocytes are known as T 'helper' (Th) cells, and form the majority of the circulating T-cell population. Their roles include the production of cytokines to promote an inflammatory response in the presence of the appropriate antigen. Such cytokines include IFNγ (from the Th1 class of CD4+ cells) and Interleukins 1, 5 and 13 (from the Th2 subset of CD4+ cells). The effects of cytokine production include activation of the monocyte/macrophage system, the promotion of granulocyte maturation and the induction of antibody synthesis by B cells.

CD8+ lymphocytes are T-suppressor/cytotoxic cells, comprising approximately one-quarter of the T cells in the peripheral blood. Their function is to destroy any cells expressing a peptide to which their TCR can bind (e.g. virally infected cells).

Natural killer cells

A small minority of mature lymphocytes are distinct from both B- and T-cell lineages. These are the NK cells, which have a role in the innate immune system, through cell-mediated cytotoxicity. NK cells differ from T cells in that they do not express TCRs, and therefore CD3, but they are nevertheless capable of mediating cell lysis. This is achieved through surface receptors that suppress NK activity when they engage self MHC molecules on a cell. However, the absence of MHC molecules on a cell removes this inhibition and the NK cells then initiate cytotoxic destruction of the target cell.

Natural killer cells express FcγRIIIA (CD16) – a receptor that recognizes antibody on the surface of a cell – and thereby induce antibody-dependent cell-mediated cytotoxicity (ADCC). Furthermore, NK cell activation leads to the production of cytokines, including IFNγ, macrophage and granulocyte-macrophage colony-stimulating factor (M-CSF, GM-CSF), IL-3 and TNFα. These cytokines effect neutrophil recruitment and function, in addition to helping to activate the monocyte–macrophage system. NK cells can lyse virus-infected cells and may be able to lyse tumour cells.

Identifying lymphoid cells in the blood and marrow

All the stages of both B- and T-cell development described above have the morphological features of either lymphoblasts or lymphocytes. The identification of different lymphocyte precursors is therefore based not on morphology but on properties including reactivity with certain monoclonal antibodies and the presence of immunoglobulin or TCR on the cell surface membrane (Tables 1.1 and 1.2). In the peripheral blood, lymphocytes may be small and compact or may appear large with azurophilic cytoplasmic granules (Figure 1.12). Such large granular lymphocytes include cytotoxic T cells and NK cells.

Table 1.1 The sequence of events during B-cell differentiation.

Characteristic	Pre-pre-B cell	Pre-B cell	Immature B cell	Mature B cell	Plasma cell
Heavy-chain genes rearranged	+	+	+	+	+
Light-chain genes rearranged	–/+	+	+	+	+
Terminal deoxynucleotidyl-transferase	+	+/–	–	–	–
Cytoplasmic μ-chains expressed	–	+	–	–	–
Surface IgM (but not IgD) expressed	–	–	+	–	–
Surface IgM and IgD expressed	–	–	–	+	–
Cytoplasmic Ig expressed	–	–	–	–	+
CD10	+	+	–	–	–
CD19	+	+	+	+	+

Ig, immunoglobulin.

Table 1.2 **The sequence of events during T-cell differentiation.**

Characteristic	Pre- T cell	Early thymocyte	Intermediate thymocyte	Late thymocyte	Mature T cell
CD7	+	+	+	+	+
Terminal deoxynucleotidyl-transferase	−/+	+	+	−	−
TCR γ genes rearranged/deleted	−	+	+	+	+
TCR β genes rearranged	−	−	+	+	+
TCR α genes rearranged	−	−	−/+	+	+
CD2	−	+	+	+	+
CD3	−	+	+	+	+
CD4 and CD8	−	−	−/+	−	−
CD4 or CD8	−	−	−	+	+

TCR, T-cell receptor.

(a) 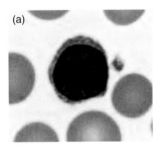 (b)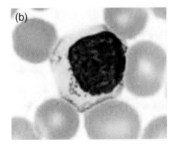

Figure 1.12 (a) A normal small lymphocyte. (b) A large lymphocyte with several azurophilic cytoplasmic granules. Large granular lymphocytes include cytotoxic T cells and natural killer (NK) cells.

Normal numbers of blood cells

The descriptions above give some sense of the way in which normal numbers of blood cells are maintained in the circulation. For red cells, this is achieved by linking the sensing of hypoxia to red cell production, while for platelets there is a balance between TPO binding to mature platelets and their bone marrow precursor, the megakaryocyte. For granulocytes, cytokine signalling related to inflammation and infection induces release from the marrow, and for lymphocytes antigenic stimulation of a pre-existing pool of lymphoid cells is key. For a healthy individual in the steady state, the numbers of each type of cell therefore exist within a predictable range. This is termed the normal or reference range, and is discussed in more detail in Chapter 2.

The non-cellular components of blood

Although the great bulk of this chapter (and the rest of the text) focuses on the function and dysfunction of blood cells, the non-cellular component also forms a key part of haematological study. Blood plasma is the liquid portion remaining following removal of blood cells by centrifugation. Principally composed of water, it also contains all the clotting factors essential for normal haemostasis (see Chapter 13); the immunoglobins synthesized and secreted by plasma cells (see Chapter 10); albumin, key for transport of some small molecules through the blood and needed to maintain oncotic pressure; and all the electrolytes, hormones and transport proteins required for the normal function of blood. Many biochemical tests are therefore performed on blood plasma (or serum, its equivalent once clotting factors have been removed).

Summary

Table 1.3 summarizes the role of each mature cell type in the peripheral blood. It is the abnormal production, function or destruction of these cells that constitutes the study of clinical haematology, which forms the basis for the rest of this book.

Table 1.3 The main functions of blood cells.

Red blood cells (erythrocytes)	Transport O_2 from lungs to tissues (see Chapters 2 and 4)
Neutrophil granulocytes	Chemotaxis, phagocytosis, killing of phagocytosed bacteria
Eosinophil granulocytes	All neutrophil functions listed above, effector cells for antibody-dependent damage to metazoal parasites, regulate immediate-type hypersensitivity reactions (inactivate histamine and leukotrienes released by basophils and mast cells)
Basophil granulocytes	Mediate immediate-type hypersensitivity (IgE-coated basophils react with specific antigen and release histamine and leukotrienes), modulate inflammatory responses by releasing heparin and proteases
Monocytes and macrophages	Chemotaxis, phagocytosis, killing of some micro-organisms, antigen presentation, release of IL-1 and TNF that stimulate bone marrow stromal cells to produce GM-CSF, G-CSF, M-CSF and IL-6
Platelets	Adhere to subendothelial connective tissue, participate in primary haemostasis
Lymphocytes	Critical for immune responses and cytokine production

G-CSF, granulocyte colony-stimulating factor; GM-CSF, granulocyte-macrophage colony-stimulating factor; Ig, immunoglobulin; IL, interleukin; M-CSF, macrophage colony-stimulating factor; TNF, tumour necrosis factor.

2

The blood count in health and disease

LEARNING OBJECTIVES

After reading this chapter, you should be able to:

✔ define and use the concept of the normal or reference range

✔ understand the variation in the blood count related to age, sex and race

✔ recognize common blood count changes in infection, inflammation, allergy and malignancy

✔ recognize and understand the emergency management of neutropenic sepsis.

Following a clinical history and physical examination, a full blood count is one of the most widely requested tests used in the investigation of disease. It is generally available in both high- and low-income countries, can be rapidly performed, and provides a broad range of information relevant to an array of haematological and non-haematological disease states.

While this text focuses on primary diseases of the blood, bone marrow and lymphoid system, the majority of changes seen in blood counts in clinical practice instead represent 'reactive' changes seen in non-haematological disease. Being able to interpret these is therefore critical for all patient-facing doctors. This chapter outlines the degree of normal variation in the blood count in healthy individuals, and discusses the changes seen in several common disease states.

What is a normal blood count?

The results of a full blood count are issued alongside a 'reference range' which gives an indication of the degree of variation that can be seen in a healthy population. Working out what constitutes this normal range usually involves sampling blood from a population of healthy volunteers and plotting the results for each parameter of the blood count. A normal distribution or bell curve is expected, and the reference range is normally given as two standard deviations from the mean of this dataset (Table 2.1).

By definition, therefore, some results outside the reference range will be found in healthy individuals, and numeric full blood count data should always be interpreted in their clinical context.

Normal variations with age, sex and race

The blood count varies throughout life in response to physiological changes, and also between groups of individuals as a consequence of hormonal or genetic differences. Neonates typically have a high haemoglobin and frequent nucleated red cells in the blood, probably explained by the relatively hypoxic conditions *in utero* while dependent on placental oxygenation. After birth, as erythropoietin levels fall (see Chapter 3), the haemoglobin gradually falls and

---

Haematology Lecture Notes, Eleventh Edition. Deborah Hay, Andrew King and Michael Desborough.
© 2023 John Wiley & Sons Ltd. Published 2023 by John Wiley & Sons Ltd.
Companion website: www.wiley.com/go/Hay/Haematology/11e

Table 2.1 **Typical normal ranges for key full blood count parameters. Note that there will be some variation in reference ranges between different clinical laboratories, related to different reagents and instruments used to generate these data.**

Parameter	Reference range
Haemoglobin	120–160 g/L (F); 130–170 g/L (M)
Mean cell volume (MCV)	82–100 fL
Mean cell haemoglobin (MCH)	27–32 pg
Red blood cell (RBC) count	$3.8–4.8 \times 10^{12}$/L
Total white blood cell (WBC) count	$4–11 \times 10^9$/L
Neutrophil count	$2–7 \times 10^9$/L
Lymphocyte count	$1–4 \times 10^9$/L
Eosinophil count	$0.0–0.5 \times 10^9$/L
Basophil count	$0.0–0.1 \times 10^9$/L
Monocyte count	$0.2–1.0 \times 10^9$/L
Platelet count	$150–400 \times 10^9$/L
Reticulocyte count	0.5–2.0% of RBCs

The effect of testosterone on erythropoiesis also influences the full blood count, with the haemoglobin, red cell count and haematocrit of postpubertal males being higher than that of adult females. Although testosterone levels fall with age, neither this nor other potential age-related changes in haematopoiesis are commonly acknowledged in the normal ranges for laboratory haematology parameters at present, though there is increasing understanding of the changes to the full blood count that arise with age (Figure 2.1).

The ethnic origin of individuals is also of significance in interpreting blood count data. The most significant aspect is the lower neutrophil count observed in many individuals of Afro-Caribbean ethnic origin. Neutrophil counts as low as 1×10^9/L are not uncommon in this context, and an awareness of this can prevent over-investigation of otherwise well individuals from the appropriate ethnic groups.

The blood count is also subject to change in pregnancy. While both the total blood volume and red cell mass increase significantly in a normal pregnancy, the blood volume increase is the greater, and a dilutional anaemia is therefore expected. A mild increase in the mean cell volume (MCV) is also typically seen, which may in part reflect the increased reticulocyte percentage in pregnant women's blood. A mild neutrophilia can be seen, reflecting the physiological stress of pregnancy, and a 'gestational thrombocytopenia' is also common – a mild decrease in platelet count due to increased platelet activation and clearance. In each case, these findings should be considered as normal variants rather than as pathological findings, emphasizing the importance of understanding the clinical context in which every blood count is taken.

nucleated red cells become much less common in circulating blood. Levels of vitamin K-dependent clotting factors are also at significantly lower levels in neonates, as the fetal liver lacks capacity efficiently to complete the γ-carboxylation of these factors. The clotting times (see Chapter 13) are therefore longer in neonates than in adulthood.

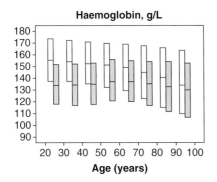 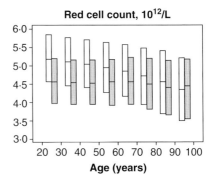

Figure 2.1 Changing levels of haemoglobin and red cell count in adults aged 20–100. White bars: men; grey bars: women.
Source: Courtesy of Dr Jacob Zierk and colleagues, University Hospital Erlangen. *British Journal of Haematology*, 2020;189: 777–789.

Typical changes in disease states

Infection, inflammation and trauma

One of the most common clinical abnormalities of the full blood count in non-specialist practice is the array of changes seen in response to acute infection and inflammation. Most striking amongst these is the development of an increased neutrophil count (neutrophilia), mediated by the effect of the cytokine granulocyte colony stimulating factor (GCSF) on the bone marrow. Bacterial infection especially is characterized by a neutrophilia. Counts ranging from 10–20 × 10^9/L are not uncommon, though severe infection or trauma may even give counts as high as 30–50 × 10^9/L. Neutrophil counts in excess of this, or without accompanying features of severe infection, should prompt investigation for conditions where there is autonomous or neoplastic production (i.e. the myeloproliferative neoplasms, see also Chapter 8).

Typical blood film features suggestive of infection include toxic granulation of neutrophils and 'left shift' – a feature describing the release of less mature neutrophil precursors from the marrow into the blood (Figure 2.2).

As neutrophils migrate from the circulation to the tissues to combat infection, prolonged infection can result in depletion of the neutrophil population and a neutropenia may be seen. The changes seen in bacterial infection are also commonly seen in non-infectious inflammation (e.g. inflammatory arthritides, vasculitis, burns) and in trauma and surgery.

While viral infection may not produce especially marked changes in the blood count, some recurrent features are seen. A lymphocytosis may be present in some viral infections, with acute Epstein–Barr virus infection being among those showing the most prominent 'reactive' lymphocytosis. The lymphocytes seen in this condition, and in other infectious mononucleosis syndromes, are large with basophilic cytoplasm and sometime azurophilic granules (Figure 2.3).

A mild neutropenia can also be seen with this clinical picture, which may sometimes raise concerns about a more significant primary haematological disorder. The monospot test (Box 2.1) is often a useful diagnostic adjunct. In older patients, a persistent lymphocytosis is more likely to indicate an underlying clonal haematological disorder, and investigation with immunophenotyping is required (see Chapter 7).

Parasitic infection produces additional blood count anomalies which are not typically seen in bacterial or viral infection, with an eosinophilia being the most prominent amongst these (Figure 2.4). This increase in eosinophils is attributed to the effect of parasite-induced IL-5 signalling on the bone marrow. A similar eosinophilia is seen in the context of allergic inflammation and atopy, including in patients with eczema and asthma, and also characterizes a range of vasculitic conditions. Rarely, an eosinophilia may be

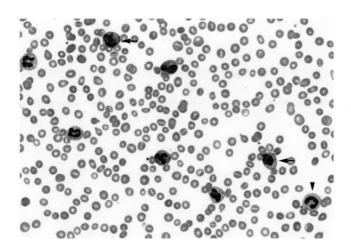

Figure 2.2 A blood film showing 'left shift' with mature neutrophils, band form neutrophil (arrowhead) and myelocytes (arrows). Teadrop poikilocytes are also present, which may suggest marrow infiltration; see below.

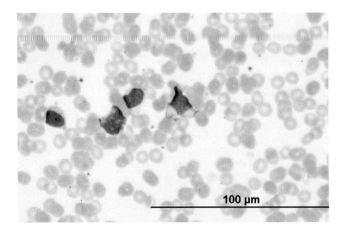

Figure 2.3 Reactive lymphocytes typical of viral infection.

Box 2.1 Monospot test

Infection with Epstein–Barr virus (EBV) gives a clinical picture of fever, pharyngitis, lymphadenopathy and often hepatosplenomegaly. Some patients also develop autoimmune complications such as autoimmune haemolytic anaemia and immune thrombocytopenia. The combination of atypical lymphoid cells on a blood film with other cytopenias and a rapidly developing lymphadenopathy can sometimes raise concerns about the possibility of high-grade lymphoma, and immediate diagnostic tests for EBV infection are therefore clinically valuable.

As well as the typical reactive lymphocytosis on the blood film, this infection is also characterized by the development of antibodies capable of agglutinating red cells of other species, such as horse or sheep, and this feature can be exploited diagnostically. Non-specific antibodies are absorbed out using guinea pig kidney cells, allowing the specific antibodies to be titrated against sheep red cells; this is the basis of the Paul–Bunnell test. The monospot test uses a similar agglutination reaction for the detection of heterophile antibodies against equine red blood cells. When positive, the monospot test is highly suggestive of infectious mononucleosis caused by EBV. While the detection of specific anti-EBV IgM antibodies remains the gold standard diagnostic test for this infection, the monospot test is readily available and gives instant results, making it a valuable test in the clinical setting.

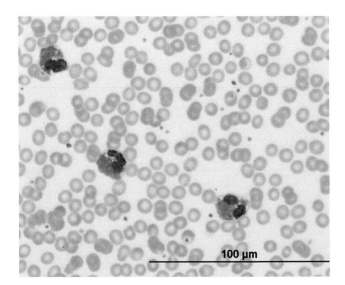

Figure 2.4 Eosinophils, typically seen in allergic/atopic states, or in response to parasitic infection.

seen in reaction to an underlying lymphoma, especially Hodgkin lymphoma or T-cell lymphomas.

Changes secondary to infection and inflammation are not limited to the leucocytes. A thrombocytosis is commonly observed in this context, and may even reach levels of >1000 × 10⁹/L. A diagnosis of primary myeloproliferative neoplasms therefore first requires careful exclusion of so-called 'reactive thrombocytoses'.

Marrow infiltration

Malignant infiltration of the bone marrow can be seen with both primary haematological cancers and metastatic disease from non-haematological primary malignancies. The former are discussed in more detail in the following chapters, but it is important to recognize that the blood count and blood film may provide the first indication of metastatic involvement of the marrow by solid malignancies. Primary tumours which commonly metastasize to the marrow include carcinoma of the breast, bronchus, kidney, thyroid and prostate. In some cases, metastatic disease may be the initial presenting feature. Anaemia is common in this context, and may be either normocytic or macrocytic. Less commonly, neutropenia or thrombocytopenia may also be seen. Figure 2.5 shows the typical appearance of the blood in a patient with metastatic carcinoma in the bone marrow; nucleated red blood cells are seen, alongside relatively immature granulocyte precursors. This combination, known as 'leucoerythroblastic change', is also seen in

severe sepsis, but requires urgent investigation in any patient in whom there is no clinical evidence of sepsis. Some of the more mature red cells also have an atypical 'teardrop' shape – this can be seen in any situation in which the bone marrow is abnormally packed, but in the context of leucoerythroblastic change may point to marrow infiltration. The bone marrow trephine shown in Figure 2.6 demonstrates the appearance of infiltration by non-haematopoietic malignancy.

Some malignancies will have additional and specific haematological complications, including disseminated intravascular coagulation and malignancy-associated thrombotic microangiopathies (see Chapter 13) and even endocrine complications such as secondary polycythaemia in the case of rare epo-secreting renal cell carcinomas, adrenal tumours and uterine tumours. The majority will manifest some degree of the anaemia of chronic disease.

Red cell changes in response to non-haematological disease

As well as falling in the context of acute or chronic haemorrhage, the red cell count is also impacted by chronic inflammation. This is discussed in Chapter 3. Reactive increases in red cell production can also be seen in the context of chronic hypoxia, and this 'secondary polycythaemia' is not uncommon in patients with severe chronic obstructive airways disease.

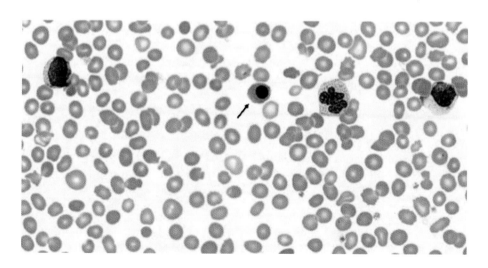

Figure 2.5 Blood film appearances with metastatic disease in the marrow. There is leucoerythroblastic change (left shift, with nucleated red blood cell, arrowed) and the red cells show variable morphology. MGG stain.

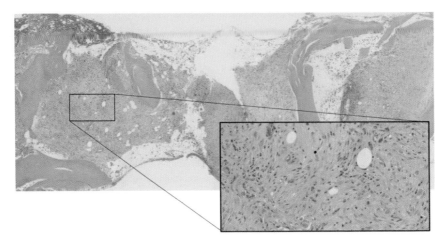

Figure 2.6 Low- and high-power views of a bone marrow biopsy infiltrated with metastatic carcinoma. Normal haematopoiesis is entirely effaced by an infiltrate of non-haematopoietic cells with associated fibrotic change.

Hypersplenism and hyposplenism

While splenomegaly is commonly the result of a primary haematological problem (e.g. a lymphoproliferative disease, myeloproliferative neoplasm or chronic haemolytic anaemia), splenomegaly of even non-haematological origin can have a striking effect on the blood count. Since blood can pool in an enlarged spleen, it is common to see a reduction in red cell, leucocyte and platelet counts in patients with splenomegaly. By contrast, a mild to moderate leucocytosis and thrombocytosis is typically seen in patients who have hyposplenism, whether this arises as a result of surgical removal of the spleen or disease affecting its function (coeliac disease and some autoimmune disorders, for example). A loss of the filtration mechanism also gives rise to classic red cell anomalies on the blood film (Figure 2.7).

From a clinical perspective, these changes are much less significant than the loss of the immunological function of the spleen – overwhelming postsplenectomy infection being a major concern for patients with reduced splenic function, since they are unable to mount an adequate response to blood-borne encapsulated bacteria.

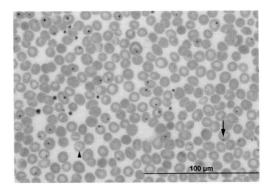

Figure 2.7 Blood film from a patient post-splenectomy. Many red cells contain small, dense darkly staining inclusions, termed Howell–Jolly bodies (arrowed). These are nuclear remnants and are normally removed by the macrophages of the spleen. Occasional target cells are also seen (arrowhead), also typical of postsplenectomy red cell change.

The effect of drugs on the blood count

Many medications have predictable and unavoidable effects on the blood count; cytotoxic chemotherapy is an example which is expected, through its normal mechanism of action, to result in significant cytopenias. In many cases, severe neutropenia and thrombocytopenia will result and patients receiving such therapy should be counselled on the risks of developing neutropenic sepsis (Box 2.2). Other drug treatments can also result in clinically important cytopenias, requiring careful counselling of patients to seek medical attention if they develop features suggestive of neutropenia (e.g. mouth ulcers, fever,

Box 2.2 Haematological emergency: neutropenic sepsis

Neutrophils are essential for the maintenance of mucosal integrity. Whether the neutropenia arises from administration of cytotoxic chemotherapy or as a result of marrow infiltration, one of the earliest clinical features is the development of mouth ulcers. These changes are not limited to the oral mucosa, however: disruption to mucosal integrity throughout the gut can result in the greater ease of ingress of Gram-negative organisms from the gut into the bloodstream, where the lack of neutrophils for the immediate innate immune response means there is a greater likelihood of overwhelming bacterial infection. For this reason, any fever in a neutropenic individual should be treated aggressively, typically with broad-spectrum intravenous antibiotics.

While antibiotic choice will be determined by local policy and culture sensitivities where known, immediate therapy with a broad-spectrum agent with good Gram-negative cover is essential in the first instance. Piperacillin-tazobactam is a typical first-line choice for most neutropenic patients who are not penicillin allergic. Careful clinical assessment for sources of infection is essential, and meticulous attention to fluid balance and cardiovascular status is also needed, as clinical deterioration can be rapid.

If the fever persists, a programme of planned progressive therapy is used, with additional antibiotics to ensure good Gram-positive cover, and also antifungal agents. Patients with prolonged neutropenia are particularly prone to develop fungal infections, notably with *Candida* and *Aspergillus*. *Candida* species usually affect the mouth and other mucosal surfaces, whereas *Aspergillus* species tend to cause invasive pulmonary disease.

Box 2.3 Causes of selective neutropenia

Physiological
Benign ethnic neutropenia in people of
  Afro-Caribbean ethnicity

Drugs
Antipsychotic medications, e.g. clozapine
Non-steroidal anti-inflammatory drugs
Disease-modifying rheumatological agents:
  methotrexate, leflunomide, gold salts
Antibacterials: chloramphenicol, co-trimoxazole
  (sulfamethoxazole-trimethoprim), other
  sulfonamides, macrolides
Some antithyroid drugs, e.g. carbimazole
Some antiepileptic drugs
Cytotoxic chemotherapy agents

Infections
Bacterial: overwhelming pyogenic infections,
  brucellosis, typhoid, miliary tuberculosis
Some viral infections, notably HIV; protozoal and
  fungal infections

Immune neutropenia
Systemic lupus erythematosus (SLE), Felty syndrome,
  autoimmune neutropenia, neonatal alloimmune
  neutropenia

Miscellaneous
Hypothyroidism, hypopituitarism, anorexia nervosa,
  cyclical neutropenia, congenital neutropenia

clinical signs of infection). The antithyroid medication carbimazole is one such example, and has been associated with the development of not just severe neutropenia but agranulocytosis (absence of all granulocytes) in a minority of patients. Some drugs have also been associated with the development of immune cytopenias, discussed further in Chapters 3 and 13. Box 2.3 highlights some drugs commonly

recognized as causing neutropenia, along with other potential causes.

Some commonly used drugs will cause a leucocytosis rather than a leucopenia. Corticosteroids are perhaps the best example, causing demargination of neutrophils from the endothelial surfaces of blood vessels into the laminar flow of the circulation, thereby resulting in a predictable neutrophilia.

3

Anaemia: general principles

LEARNING OBJECTIVES

After reading this chapter, you should be able to:

- ✔ define anaemia and recognize its clinical signs and symptoms
- ✔ understand the mechanisms by which anaemia may arise
- ✔ classify anaemia by reticulocyte response and/or by red cell size
- ✔ suggest causes of microcytic, normocytic and macrocytic anaemia
- ✔ describe normal iron metabolism, how iron deficiency may arise, and how to investlgate it
- ✔ describe how iron overload occurs
- ✔ understand the pathophysiology and typical laboratory features of the anaemia of chronic disease
- ✔ describe megaloblastic anaemia and the role of vitamin B12 and folate in red cell production
- ✔ appreciate the differences between normoblastic and megaloblastic anaemia
- ✔ explain how the failure of the normal control of red cell production can lead to polycythaemia.

Anaemia is one of the most common haematological abnormalities, affecting around one-third of the world's population. Its clinical importance cannot be overstated, as it is associated increased morbidity and mortality, poor birth outcomes, problems with cognitive development in children, and reduced work productivity in adults. It is also a sensitive marker of general health, and is frequently the prompt to further investigation in the diagnosis of a wide range of haematological and non-haematological disorders.

Anaemia is defined as a haemoglobin (Hb) level below the normal range. This normal range will vary between individuals of different ages and sexes, reflecting differences in the normal process of erythropoiesis in different physiological situations. (Table 3.1; see Chapter 2). These differences must be taken into account when interpreting the full blood count and assessing the potential causes and significance of anaemia.

Haematology Lecture Notes, Eleventh Edition. Deborah Hay, Andrew King and Michael Desborough.

Table 3.1 Reference ranges for haemoglobin (Hb) values.

	Hb concentration (g/L)
Cord blood	135–205
First day of life	150–235
Children, 6 months–6 years	110–145
Children, 6–14 years	120–155
Adult males	130–170
Adult females (non-pregnant)	120–160
Pregnant females	110–140

Defining the presence of anaemia in a patient is only the start – anaemia is not a diagnosis in itself. In every case, it is essential to seek an explanation for it in order to address the underlying cause and provide appropriate treatment.

Symptoms and signs of anaemia

The clinical features of anaemia vary depending on how rapidly the anaemia develops. Most cases of anaemia caused by nutritional deficiencies, for example, are of gradual onset, and physiological adaptations mean the associated symptoms are relatively mild. Mechanisms such as an increase in red cell 2,3-diphosphoglycerate (2,3-DPG), which shifts the oxygen dissociation curve to the right and permits enhanced delivery of O_2 in the tissues (see Chapter 5), can compensate for small reductions in haemoglobin. Cardiovascular adaptive mechanisms, such as increased stroke volume and heart rate, are also deployed, though these may be limited in older patients with impaired cardiovascular reserve. This situation contrasts with that seen in anaemia of acute onsent (e.g. acute haemorrhage or acquired haemolytic anaemia), where the lack of time to develop physiological adaptation means that symptoms arise at a less marked level of anaemia.

Typical symptoms of anaemia include lassitude, fatigue, dyspnoea on exertion, palpitations and headache; older patients with impaired cardiovascular reserve may also develop angina and intermittent claudication. Physical signs include pallor of the skin and/or conjunctiva, tachycardia, flow murmurs and, in severe cases, congestive cardiac failure. Clues to the underlying aetiology of anaemia must also be sought in the clinical history and examination.

Normal control of red cell production

In healthy adults, there is a steady-state equilibrium between the rate of release of new red cells from the bone marrow into the circulation and the removal of senescent red cells from the circulation by macrophages. The renally secreted hormone erythropoietin (epo) is the main agent responsible for translating tissue hypoxia into increased red cell production to maintain this balance (see also Chapter 1).

For anaemia to arise, there must be either a failure of adequate production of red cells (e.g. insufficient erythroid tissue in the marrow or poor-quality erythroid maturation) or an increased rate of red cell loss (perhaps through blood loss or haemolysis) as shown in Box 3.1. The reticulocyte count is a useful marker to enable differentiation of anaemia caused by failure of production from that caused by accelerated red cell destruction. If epo is able to drive additional red cell

---

Box 3.1 Mechanisms leading to anaemia

- Blood loss
- Decreased red cell lifespan (haemolytic anaemia):
  - Congenital defect (e.g. sickle cell disease, hereditary spherocytosis)
  - Acquired defect (e.g. immune mechanisms, malaria, some drugs)
- Impairment of red cell formation:
  - Insufficient erythropoiesis
  - Ineffective erythropoiesis
- Pooling and destruction of red cells in an enlarged spleen
- Increased plasma volume (splenomegaly, pregnancy)

production in response to anaemia – which will require the normal processes of red cell formation to be intact – the reticulocyte count will be high. Therefore, where the primary abnormality leading to anaemia is a shortened red cell survival or direct loss of red cells through haemorrhage, the reticulocyte count will be increased. Bone marrow failure syndromes, by contrast, will have a low reticulocyte count, as will any acquired limitation on the marrow's ability to produce red blood cells, such as haematinic deficiency. In many cases of anaemia, however, both mechanisms have a role; in anaemia caused by chronic bleeding from the gastrointestinal tract, for example, red cells are lost from the circulation, while the development of iron deficiency prevents an adequate bone marrow response. Similarly, haemolytic conditions, which are typically associated with a reticulocytosis, may be complicated by the development of folate deficiency; this will impede the bone marrow response and may come to limit the expected reticulocytosis.

Thus, although the reticulocyte count is an important part of the assessment of any patient with anaemia, it may not be straightforward to interpret.

Morphological classification of anaemias

An alternative and very widely used strategy for thinking about anaemia is to classify it in terms of red cell size. Characteristic changes in the size of red cells (mean cell volume, MCV), and their degree of haemoglobinization (mean cell haemoglobin, MCH), accompany the development of anaemia of different aetiologies, and can be used to divide anaemia into three main groups.

- Microcytic hypochromic (low MCV and low MCH).
- Macrocytic (high MCV).
- Normocytic (normal MCV).

A summary of this classification is shown in Table 3.2. Anaemia resulting from iron deficiency is typically microcytic and hypochromic, though the precise mechanisms by which microcytosis arises remain incompletely understood. The thalassaemias are also typically microcytic hypochromic anaemias. By contrast, anaemia resulting from vitamin B12 or folate deficiency, in which there is a

Table 3.2 Morphological classification of anaemia.

Type	MCV (fL)[a]	Causes
Microcytic	<82	Iron deficiency, thalassaemia syndromes, some long-standing cases of anaemia of chronic disease
Normocytic	82–99	Acute blood loss, some cases of anaemia of chronic disease, chronic kidney disease, some haemolytic anaemias, leucoerythroblastic anaemias
Macrocytic	>100	Alcohol excess, folate deficiency, vitamin B12 deficiency

[a]Note that normal ranges will change from laboratory to laboratory, and local ranges must always be used to interpret results.

failure of nuclear maturation and disrupted cell division, is classically macrocytic. Haemolytic anaemias characterized by a brisk reticulocytosis may also have a slightly higher MCV, since reticulocytes tend to be larger than mature red cells. Normocytic anaemias include those caused by acute blood loss, where there has not been time to produce a significant marrow response.

However, the morphological classification of anaemia is not always so readily interpreted. Some conditions can straddle two categories; the anaemia of chronic disease, for example, may be either normocytic or microcytic, with the MCV typically falling in patients who have especially prolonged periods of anaemia. Similarly, anaemia with two contributing mechanisms may produce results that are harder to interpret; for example, in coeliac disease there may be a combined deficiency of iron and folic acid, with each blunting the other's effect on the MCV to produce a normocytic anaemia. Nevertheless, the classification of anaemia by MCV does have the merit of highlighting the most frequently seen and readily treated causes of anaemia: haematinic deficiencies (lack of iron, B12 or folate).

A more detailed discussion of the most common causes of anaemia is found in the following sections, and Figure 3.1 shows the classic appearances of red cells in these conditions.

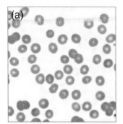 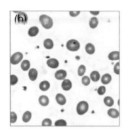 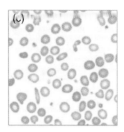

Figure 3.1 Normal and abnormal red cells. (a) Normochromic, normocytic cells. The red cell should normally be approximately the same size as the nucleus of a small lymphocyte, and the cell should have an area of central pallor of approximately one-third its diameter. (b) Oval macrocytes, in a patient with B12 deficiency. (c) Hypochromic, microcytic cells in a patient with iron deficiency. Many of the red cells have only a thin rim of haemoglobin and some are very small. Pencil cells are also seen. All with MGG stain, at high-power magnification.

Microcytic anaemia: iron handling abnormalities and iron deficiency anaemia

Iron deficiency anaemia is thought to be the most common cause of anaemia worldwide. This section outlines the normal processes of iron metabolism, essential for an appreciation of how iron deficiency arises and is managed. The consequences of deranged iron absorption and iron overload are also described (Box 3.2).

Iron absorption

Excess iron is potentially toxic. Therefore, because the body has no physiological mechanism for upregulating iron excretion, its absorption from the gut is tightly controlled. This permits iron absorption to be maximized when stores are low or when there is a need to increase erythropoiesis, but minimizes the risk of excess iron absorption when stores are already adequate.

The normal Western diet contains 10–20 mg of iron per day, of which typically 5–10% is absorbed. Normally, iron in the duodenum is reduced to its ferrous (Fe^{2+}) form by duodenal cytochrome b, before binding the divalent metal transporter 1 (DMT1) on the apical (luminal) membrane of the duodenal enterocyte. Iron taken up into the cell in this way is either stored directly as ferritin (which may be lost with desquamation of the enterocyte from the lumen of the gut) or oxidized to the ferric form by the trans-membrane protein hephaestin and transported to the plasma via the molecule ferroportin on the basolateral membrane of the enterocyte. Iron in the plasma is bound to the transport protein transferrin, which delivers iron to the bone marrow for erythropoiesis. Here it enters the erythroid cells by interacting with the surface transferrin receptor 1.

At the end of their lifespan, red cells are removed from the circulation by macrophages especially within the spleen, and have their haem moiety recycled. The iron is released from the haem ring and bound to transferrin to be redelivered to the bone marrow, or stored as ferritin. This process is summarized in Figure 3.2.

Several checkpoints operate during this process. The uptake of iron into the duodenal enterocyte may be affected by the local oxygen tension, mediated by the effect of the transcription factor hypoxia inducible factor (HIF) on the expression of DMT1. The production of DMT1 is also influenced directly by iron: iron affects the binding of iron-response proteins to iron-response elements in the 5′ untranslated region of the mRNA for this gene, determining the rate of its translation.

Once iron is inside the enterocyte, its transfer to the circulation is controlled by the hormone hepcidin. This protein, produced by the liver, binds to ferroportin and induces its internalization. This prevents the efflux of iron from the enterocyte, such that it will be lost when the cell is desquamated into the lumen of the gut. Hepcidin therefore provides a key mechanism for determining how much iron is absorbed from the gut.

Hepcidin expression is itself regulated directly by several mechanisms relevant to the assessment of iron stores. When carrying iron, transferrin is involved

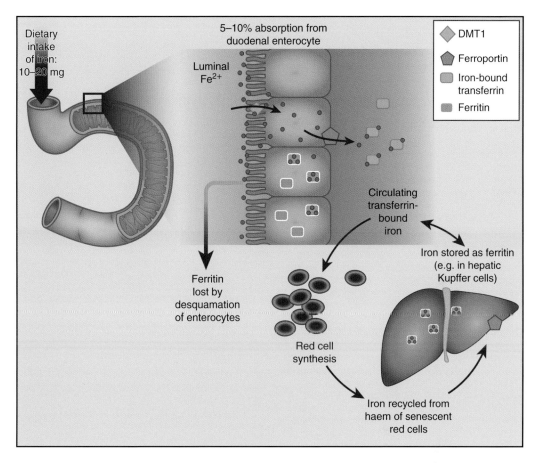

Figure 3.2 A summary of iron handling. Note that there is no physiological mechanism to enhance iron loss after it is absorbed from the duodenal enterocytes. Hepcidin, produced by the liver when iron replete, influences the production and/or function of key molecules in iron absorption, including ferroportin, divalent metal transporter 1 (DMT1) and transferrin.

in a signalling pathway that enhances hepcidin expression, thus reducing iron absorption from the gut. By contrast, HIF is able to contribute to a decrease in hepcidin expression, as can enhanced erythropoietic activity (Box 3.2). In these two circumstances, a reduction in hepcidin will result in increased iron absorption in settings in which additional iron absorption is likely to be beneficial. A further interface between inflammation and hepcidin expression is critical for the development of the anaemia of chronic disease – discussed further below.

In short, although adults who have normal iron stores absorb approximately 5–10% of their total intake (0.5–2 mg/day), this is subject to great variation in response to physiological demand. Hepcidin is the master regulator of this process. Normally, in the setting of iron loading, hepcidin expression is upregulated and iron absorption is limited; where there is a requirement for increased erythroid activity, hepcidin levels fall and more iron absorption is permitted. Clearly, there are situations in which these signals conflict with each other – for example, in the thalassaemias, when anaemia and iron loading coexist (see Box 3.2 and Chapter 5). Here, pharmacological means of iron control must be employed.

How does iron deficiency arise?

Iron deficiency will arise in any of three settings:

- A diet containing too little iron to meet physiological needs.
- Malabsorption of iron from the duodenum.
- Increased loss of iron (e.g. through haemorrhage).

Box 0.2 Iron overload

Iron absorption from a normal diet is inappropriately increased in hereditary haemochromatosis, a collection of conditions in which there are defects in the key proteins responsible for iron regulation. In each case, there is a failure of adequate downregulation of ferroportin by hepcidin, leading to uncontrolled iron transition from the enterocyte to the circulation. If the ability of transferrin to bind iron is saturated, non-transferrin-bound iron is found in the circulation; this form may be taken up by many cell types, including hepatocytes and cardiac myocytes, where it has a damaging oxidant effect.

The most common form is *HFE* haemochromatosis, an autosomal recessive condition with an incidence of 5 per 1000 in northern European populations. Most patients have a point mutation leading to the amino substitution C282Y in the *HFE* gene; others have compound heterozygosity for mutations leading to the substitutions C282Y and H63D. The *HFE* gene is thought to have a key role in the control of hepatic synthesis of hepcidin, and homozygotes usually develop symptoms from tissue damage from severe iron overload between the ages of 40 and 60 years. In women, the regular loss of iron during menstruation typically delays the age of onset of iron loading. Iron deposition occurs in several organs, and haemochromatosis may eventually cause cardiac dysfunction, cirrhosis, diabetes mellitus, testicular atrophy and skin pigmentation if untreated. However, the textbook clinical description of 'bronze diabetes' is now uncommon, with most patients being diagnosed either incidentally or when presenting with non-specific symptoms such as fatigue. Family screening is also undertaken for first degree relatives of any individual diagnosed with haemochromatosis.

In addition to the haemochromatosis caused by *HFE* mutations, other forms exist, caused by mutations affecting the ferroportin gene and the transferrin receptor gene. However, these are much less common.

Iron loading can also occur when there are conflicting signals regarding the body's iron requirements. Consider patients with thalassaemia (see Chapter 5) in whom iron stores are not reduced, but in whom ineffective erythropoiesis leads to a persistent erythroid signal to suppress hepcidin expression and increase iron absorption. The protein erythroferrone, secreted by early erythroid precursors which are increased in number in ineffective erythropoiesis, has been found to be responsible for this effect. In this clinical setting, excess iron absorption from the gastrointestinal tract is compounded by iron entering the body through transfusions, and severe iron loading can result.

Whatever the cause, estimations of the extent of iron loading can be made from the serum ferritin. Liver biopsy remains the gold standard for quantifying iron levels accurately, and will also assess the extent of hepatic damage caused by iron excess; however, specialist magnetic resonance imaging (MRI) protocols are now widely available and permit a non-invasive method for examining iron overload. T2* MRI is an excellent method for assessing cardiac iron loading and Ferriscan™ is widely used for assessment of hepatic iron loading.

Where possible, treatment is by venesection. However, venesection is clearly inappropriate in patients who develop iron overload because of ineffective erythropoiesis and chronic transfusion programmes. Here the use of iron chelators is needed (see also Chapter 5).

Iron deficiency is not uncommon in infants who are given unsupplemented milk or who are exclusively breast fed for more than 6 months. Similarly, the increased iron requirements of growing children and menstruating women can also put them at risk of iron deficiency. As the physiological requirements for iron rise substantially during pregnancy, iron deficiency is common then too, even in the context of a good diet. Iron is most readily absorbed in its haem form, as non-haem iron may be bound by phytates and phosphates also found in food. Vegetarian diets, containing principally non-haem iron, may therefore also predispose to dietary iron deficiency.

Gastric HCl is needed to reduce ferric to ferrous iron for efficient absorption. Therefore, partial or complete gastrectomy can cause iron deficiency through lack of HCl (achlorhydria). Certain antacid compounds have been described as having a similar effect, though long-term treatment with proton pump inhibitors such as omeprazole appears to be implicated in iron deficiency only very rarely. Duodenal pathology such as coeliac disease may also inhibit the absorption of iron from an adequate diet.

However, blood loss remains the most frequent cause of iron deficiency. In women of child-bearing age, menorrhagia must be considered; in postmenopausal women and in men, gastrointestinal bleeding is the most likely explanation, and an unexplained finding of iron deficiency should prompt a careful evaluation for gastric and colonic pathology, including malignancies.

These causes are summarized in Box 3.3.

Manifestations of iron deficiency

Although iron is found in every cell (e.g. as part of cofactors for the enzymes of the respiratory chain), at any time the bulk of iron in a healthy individual is found in red cells. Haematological manifestations are therefore among the first seen in iron deficiency.

If iron deficiency is mild, there will simply be a depletion of iron stores. This may be entirely without clinical consequence. However, as the supply of iron to the tissues is hampered, the red cells will develop hypochromic microcytic features. As deficiency progresses, the haemoglobin falls, giving a hypochromic microcytic anaemia. Other tissues are also affected in severe iron deficiency: there may be angular stomatitis, brittle and misshapen nails (including the classic but rarely seen spoon-shaped nails, koilonychia) and dysphagia in some cases associated with a pharyngeal stricture or web. Rarely, some patients also manifest bizarre dietary cravings, known as pica.

The blood film will show characteristic features; in addition to the hypochromic, microcytic red cells, there may be misshapen red cells (poikilocytes), including pencil cells and target cells. These are shown in Figure 3.3. The inability of the bone marrow to respond adequately will result in a reticulocyte count lower than expected for the degree of anaemia.

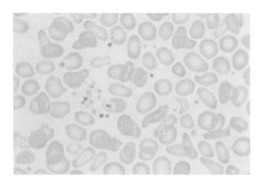

Figure 3.3 Peripheral blood film from a patient with untreated iron deficiency anaemia. Hypochromic microcytes and elongated ('pencil-shaped') poikilocytes are present.

Confirming a diagnosis of iron deficiency

While the combination of a microcytic hypochromic anaemia with a likely history may strongly suggest iron deficiency, confirmation is still required. The key laboratory parameters of iron status are the serum ferritin, transferrin and serum iron levels. While none is a perfect indicator of iron status, all three together permit the best estimation of iron status short of invasive tests like bone marrow biopsy.

Ferritin is the main storage protein for iron and for concentrations <1000 μg/L it roughly correlates with the amount of tissue storage iron. As might be predicted, ferritin levels are typically low in iron deficiency (Table 3.3). However, there is no single value for ferritin concentration that clearly separates individuals with good iron stores from those without, and there is a considerable overlap in ferritin levels between these two groups. In the study illustrated in Figure 3.4, all women with ferritin levels below 14 μg/L were iron deficient, but 25% of the iron-deficient women had ferritin levels above this value. This discrepancy arises because ferritin is also an acute-phase reactant, which is typically raised in infection and inflammation. Thus, normal serum ferritin levels may be found in the presence of reduced iron stores in acute and chronic infections and in malignancy.

Serum iron also falls in the context of iron deficiency, but there are often marked diurnal and day-to-day changes in serum iron concentration. Along with recognized reductions in the serum iron concentration in the context of infection and inflammation, this makes it an unreliable indicator of iron status when assayed alone.

Table 3.3 Typical iron studies in people with normal iron stores, individuals with iron depletion without anaemia, and in iron deficiency anaemia, while uncomplicated by inflammation.

	Normal iron stores	Depleted iron stores		
		Without reduction of iron supply to tissues	Reduced iron supply to tissues, no anaemia	Iron deficiency anaemia
Serum ferritin (µg/L)	Normal	Normal	Low	Low
Transferrin (g/L)	Normal	Normal or raised	Normal or raised	Typically raised
Serum iron (µmol/L)	Normal	Normal	Low	Low
Transferrin saturation (%)	Normal	Normal	Low	Low
Hb concentration	Normal	Normal	Within reference range	Below reference range

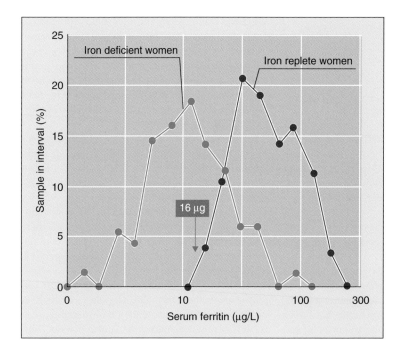

Figure 3.4 The distribution of the serum ferritin concentration in 105 women with stainable iron in the bone marrow (●) and 69 women with no stainable iron (●). *Source*: Hallberg *et al.* (1993) Screening for iron deficiency: an analysis based on bone-marrow examinations and serum ferritin determinations in a population sample of women. *British Journal of Haematology*, 85(4): 787–798. Reproduced with permission of John Wiley and Sons.

However, serum iron can also be interpreted in the context of the transferrin concentration, to give a measure of transferrin saturation (iron/transferrin × 100). Transferrin, synthesized in the liver, is generally increased in states of iron deficiency; along with the reduced serum iron, this leads to a reduction in transferrin saturation. A transferrin saturation of <20% generally represents iron depletion, while levels >45%

suggest iron loading. (Some laboratories provide equivalent data in the form of the total iron-binding capacity, TIBC.) However, as with ferritin, factors other than iron status can have an impact on transferrin levels. Chronic liver disease and chronic inflammatory states will cause the transferrin level to fall, while its production is often increased in women taking the oral contraceptive pill.

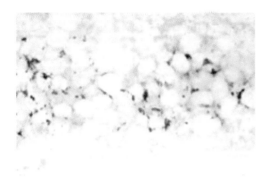

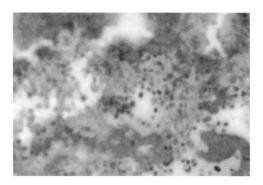

Figure 3.5 Marrow fragment containing normal quantities of storage iron. The haemosiderin stains blue (Perls' acid ferrocyanide stain).

Figure 3.6 Marrow fragment from a patient with iron deficiency anaemia showing an absence of storage iron (Perls' acid ferrocyanide stain). Contrast with Figure 3.5.

A less readily available test is estimation of the soluble transferrin receptor concentration. The expression of the transferrin receptor on cells' plasma membranes is regulated by iron availability. Both the transmembrane form and a cleaved soluble form are increased in iron deficiency and in other conditions that give rise to erythroid hyperplasia, but they are not affected in the anaemia of chronic disease.

Newer tests, now often provided as part of the full blood count data set, include the percentage of hypochromic red cells, often a useful mark of iron deficiency when standard iron studies are made difficult to assess by concomitant inflammation. Reticulocyte haemoglobin content may also be used as a marker of iron status in some specialized contexts.

The gold standard test of iron status, undertaken when uncertainty still exists despite testing each of the above, is to stain a bone marrow aspirate with Perls' Prussian blue stain. This will highlight insoluble iron stores in the marrow; these would be absent in iron deficiency anaemia (compare Figures 3.5 and 3.6). In most clinical situations, however, a trial of oral iron supplementation and careful assessment of the haematological response may be more appropriate than a bone marrow biopsy. A good response (e.g. 10 g/L increase in Hb within 2 weeks) would provide strong support for a diagnosis of iron deficiency, even in the setting of equivocal iron studies.

Treating iron deficiency

It is important to address the underlying cause of iron deficiency. If there is gastrointestinal bleeding, its source should be found and treated; malabsorption resulting from coeliac disease should be con-

trolled. Oral iron supplementation should then be effective. Ferrous sulfate 200 mg once per day is a typical dosing regimen, though some patients find oral iron supplements difficult to tolerate as a consequence of gastrointestinal side-effects. Continuing this treatment for 3 months after the normalization of haemoglobin levels will allow replenishment of iron stores. A reticulocytosis is expected in response to treatment, with a rise in the haemoglobin level of 20 g/L over 3 weeks.

For patients who cannot tolerate any form of iron orally and for those with a severe malabsorption syndrome, parenteral iron preparations exist. These include iron sucrose, ferric carboxymaltose, ferric derisomaltose and iron dextran. All of these provide a much larger iron load per dose than would be achieved with oral iron supplementation, and several can deliver 'total dose replacement' in a single treatment episode. Most are very well tolerated, with infusion reactions and hypersensitivity reactions being rare.

As described above, the management of the iron-deficient patient is incomplete without a careful assessment of the likely underlying cause.

Other causes of microcytic hypochromic anaemia

These are shown in Box 3.1. Thalassaemia is the main differential diagnosis of iron deficiency anaemia. It is discussed in more detail in Chapter 5.

Other causes of microcytic hypochromic anaemia are rare, but include sideroblastic anaemia. Sideroblasts are red cell precursors with a perinuclear ring of coarse iron-containing mitochondria (Figures 3.7 and 3.8). This condition may be found either as an inherited (usually X-linked) or an acquired form. The common form of X-linked sideroblastic anaemia is caused by mutations in the erythroid-specific δ-aminolaevulinate synthase (*ALAS2*) gene. This encodes the enzyme catalysing the first step in haem synthesis. Pyridoxal phosphate is required for both enzyme activity and enzyme stability, and some patients with sideroblastic anaemia respond to high doses of pyridoxine given orally. The acquired condition is seen in some cases of myelodysplasia (see Chapter 8) and may also be secondary to excessive alcohol consumption, certain drugs (e.g. isoniazid or chloramphenicol) and lead poisoning.

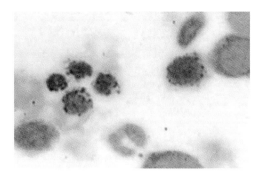

Figure 3.7 Marrow smear from a patient with primary acquired sideroblastic anaemia, stained by the Perls' acid ferrocyanide method (Prussian blue reaction). The erythroblasts contain several coarse blue–black iron-containing granules, arranged around the nucleus.

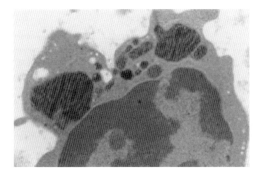

Figure 3.8 Electron micrograph of part of a ring sideroblast showing very electron-dense material between the cristae of enlarged mitochondria.

Normocytic anaemia

Anaemia of chronic disease

The anaemia of chronic disease (ACD), also known as the anaemia of inflammation, is among the most common causes of normocytic anaemia. It is associated with chronic inflammatory conditions (e.g. inflammatory arthritis), chronic infections and malignancies, and its pathogenesis is complex.

An increase in hepcidin levels is central to the development of the anaemia of chronic disease, through the effect of inflammatory cytokines including interleukin 6 (IL-6) and tumour necrosis factor α (TNFα) on hepcidin synthesis. This evolutionary mechanism for sequestering iron away from infectious microorganisms has the additional unwanted effect of limiting the availability of iron for erythropoiesis in chronic non-infectious inflammatory conditions. As well as limiting iron absorption from the gut, the increased hepcidin levels will reduce the amount of stored iron that is released from macrophages and made available for erythropoiesis (because the release of iron from these cells uses the same mechanism needed for the export of iron from enterocytes). Thus, although patients with ACD are not technically iron deficient, they are unable to make use of stored iron, giving a picture of *functional* iron deficiency.

However, the pathogenesis of ACD is more complex than the mishandling of iron alone. The activation of macrophages in the underlying chronic condition results in a reduced red cell lifespan, and this is compounded by an insufficient response from the marrow in terms of enhanced erythropoiesis. Signalling through the erythropoietin receptor appears blunted when contrasted to anaemia of other aetiologies, and the response to exogenous erythropoietin is also limited.

While the red cells in ACD are most often normocytic and normochromic, in 30–35% of patients they are hypochromic and microcytic, a picture seen especially in long-standing ACD. However, differences in the pattern of iron handling usually help in the distinction between anaemia of chronic disease and iron deficiency. In both conditions, the serum iron concentration is low, but while iron deficiency is characterized by a low serum ferritin and high transferrin, ACD tends to have a normal or even high ferritin and low transferrin. If the diagnosis from the peripheral blood tests is still in doubt, the presence or absence of storage iron in the marrow can be determined: iron stores are normal or increased in ACD and absent in iron deficiency anaemia. Pragmatically, an assessment of the clinical response to iron supplementation may be required where uncertainty persists.

Other causes of normocytic anaemia

As shown in Table 3.2, these include acute blood loss; marrow infiltration, for example by malignancy; and the anaemia associated with chronic renal disease, which is caused by a reduction in erythropoietin secretion in response to hypoxaemia.

It is important to recognize that many patients will have anaemia with contributions from more than one of these mechanisms. Dissecting the principal reasons for a patient's anaemia can therefore be far from straightforward, and empirical approaches to treatment are sometimes needed.

Macrocytic anaemia

Macrocytic anaemias can be divided into those showing megaloblastic erythropoiesis and those with normoblastic erythropoiesis. Megaloblastic erythropoiesis describes abnormal red cell development characterized by a lack of synchrony between the maturation of the red cell nucleus and its cytoplasm. It arises as a consequence of disordered DNA synthesis and results in a macrocytic anaemia, often with reduced granulocyte and platelet production in addition. Normoblastic erythropoiesis describes the normal appearance of red cell maturation, but may still be associated with a macrocytosis in the peripheral blood. Key causes in both categories are discussed below.

Causes of megaloblastic anaemia: vitamin B12 and folate deficiency

Folic acid is required for several enzymatic reactions in the body, but among the most important is the conversion of deoxyuridylate to deoxythymidylate, an essential step for the synthesis of thymidine, one of the pyrimidine bases in DNA. Without folic acid, DNA synthesis is hampered.

Vitamin B12 (cobalamin) is required for two enzymatic reactions in the body. In the first, cobalamin is a cofactor for the conversion of methylmalonyl coenzyme A (CoA) into succinyl CoA, allowing the breakdown products of certain amino acids to enter the Krebs cycle. The second reaction is a methyltransferase reaction, which converts homocysteine to methionine (by adding a methyl group) and 5-methyl tetrahydrofolate to tetrahydrofolate (by removing a methyl group). Again, cobalamin is a cofactor. One of the consequences of vitamin B12 deficiency is therefore a failure to regenerate tetrahydrofolate – and it is this form of folate that is critical for the pyrimidine synthesis step described above.

The consequences of B12 and folate deficiency can therefore be seen to overlap. Both will have a detrimental impact on DNA synthesis, and the earliest manifestations of deficiency are often seen in the blood as a consequence of the high rate of cellular proliferation in the bone marrow.

How do B12 and folate deficiency arise?

Folate is derived from many food sources, both animal and vegetable, with green leafy vegetables providing some of the richest sources (Table 3.4). The Western diet usually contains adequate quantities of folate, though deficiency because of poor intake can be seen especially in frail elderly people and in the context of alcohol excess. In some physiological circumstances, such as pregnancy and lactation, requirements markedly increase and can result in deficiency; some disease states can have a similar effect on folate requirements (through an increase in red cell production in chronic haemolytic states, or increased desquamation in psoriasis, for example). Absorption is principally from the duodenum and jejunum; coeliac disease may therefore significantly impair absorption. However, there are usually sufficient hepatic stores of folate to last for 5 or 6 months if folate intake ceased (Box 3.4).

Vitamin B12 is found exclusively in food of animal origin (see Table 3.4). On reaching the stomach, B12 is cleaved from food proteins by HCl and then bound to proteins similar to those that are responsible for its binding in the plasma – known as haptocorrins. Thus bound, B12 passes to the duodenum, where it is cleaved from the haptocorrin and binds to the glycoprotein intrinsic factor (IF). IF is essential for B12 absorption. It is highly resistant to enzymatic digestion and is able to transport B12 to the ileum, where the B12–IF complex binds its receptor, cubilin, and is endocytosed. Once passed into the circulation, B12 is bound to the transport protein transcobalamin.

Table 3.4 Key features of vitamin B12 and folate nutrition and absorption.

	Vitamin B12	Folate
Dietary sources	Only foods of animal origin	Most foods, especially green vegetables and yeast; destroyed by cooking
Average daily intake[a]	5 µg	400 µg
Minimum daily requirement[a]	1–3 µg	100–200 µg[b]
Body stores[a]	3–5 mg, mainly in the liver	8–20 mg, mainly in the liver
Time to develop deficiency in the absence of intake or absorption[a]	Anaemia in 2–10 years	Macrocytosis in 5 months
Requirements for absorption	Intrinsic factor secreted by gastric parietal cells	Conversion of polyglutamates to monoglutamates by intestinal folate conjugase
Main site of absorption	Terminal ileum	Duodenum and jejunum

[a]In adults.

[b]Higher during pregnancy and lactation.

Box 3.4 Causes of folate deficiency

- Inadequate dietary intake
- Malabsorption: coeliac disease, jejunal resection, tropical sprue
- Increased requirement: pregnancy, prematurity, chronic haemolytic anaemias
- Increased loss: long-term dialysis, congestive heart failure, acute liver disease
- Complex mechanisms: anticonvulsant therapy,[a] alcohol excess

[a]Only some cases with macrocytosis are folate deficient.

From the outline above, it is evident that vitamin B12 deficiency might arise from several mechanisms. First, unsupplemented vegan diets will lack B12. Any

Box 3.5 Mechanisms and causes of vitamin B12 deficiency

- Inadequate intake: unsupplemented vegan diet
- Inadequate secretion of intrinsic factor:
  - Pernicious anaemia
  - Total or partial gastrectomy
  - Congenital intrinsic factor deficiency (rare)
- Inadequate release of B12 from food: partial gastrectomy, vagotomy, gastritis, acid-suppressing drugs, alcohol abuse
- Diversion of dietary B12: abnormal intestinal bacterial flora, multiple jejunal diverticula, small intestinal strictures, stagnant intestinal loops
- *Diphyllobothrium latum* competition for B12
- Malabsorption: Crohn's disease, ileal resection, chronic tropical sprue
- Defective cobalamin metabolism caused by prolonged inhalation of nitrous oxide (either as a recreational drug or as anaesthetic).
- Rare genetic disorders of cobalamin deficiency (e.g. transcobalamin deficiency)

condition that results in achlorhydria (e.g. partial gastrectomy) will limit the cleavage of B12 from food-associated peptides and will also limit the availability of B12 for absorption. Disease in the terminal ileum may prevent the B12–IF complex being taken up into enterocytes, while overgrowth of gut bacteria (or the presence of the fish tapeworm, *Diphyllobothrium latum*) can 'compete' for B12 in the gut and minimize the vitamin available for absorption.

However, perhaps the best known of the conditions leading to failure of B12 absorption is pernicious anaemia. This condition arises when autoantibodies interfere with the production or function of intrinsic factor – with antiparietal cell antibodies being associated with gastric atrophy and failure of IF secretion, or anti-intrinsic factor antibodies preventing the formation of the B12–IF complex or interfering with its ability to bind to cubilin. The causes of B12 deficiency are summarized in Box 3.5.

Clinical manifestations of B12 and folate deficiency

As well as the clinical effects of a macrocytic anaemia, with possible neutropenia and thrombocytopenia if severe, deficiencies of B12 and folate will occasionally produce a mild jaundice as destruction of poorly matured erythroid precursors releases the haem

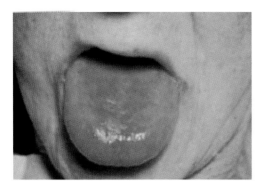

Figure 3.9 Glossitis in a woman with severe pernicious anaemia.

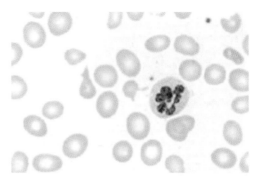

Figure 3.10 Blood film from a patient with pernicious anaemia showing oval macrocytes, other poikilocytes and a hypersegmented neutrophil.

breakdown product bilirubin (see also Chapter 4 on haemolysis).

Folate deficiency has an important relationship with neural tube defects (e.g. spina bifida) in the developing fetus, and folate supplementation is therefore given to pregnant women to reduce the risk of these congenital defects.

In addition, B12 deficiency is well known to produce a range of neurological symptoms, with a peripheral neuropathy (particularly affecting proprioception and vibration sense) being followed by demyelination of the dorsal and lateral columns of the spinal cord. This produces a clinical picture with increased tone, extensor plantars and sensory ataxia, termed subacute combined degeneration of the cord (SACD). Unlike the haematological consequences of B12 deficiency, the neurological effects may be irreversible. The precise mechanism of demyelination in SACD has not been established, but dysfunction of homocysteine methyltransferase is thought to be central to the pathophysiology.

Additional tissues that may be affected include the gastrointestinal tract (from the mouth to the colon; Figure 3.9) and the skin – all tissues characterized by high cell turnover.

Confirming a diagnosis of B12 or folate deficiency

Both B12 and folate deficiency will cause a macrocytic anaemia with megaloblastic erythropoiesis. The blood film will show oval macrocytes and hypersegmented neutrophils (again a consequence of delayed nuclear maturation; Figure 3.10). The reticulocyte count is likely to be low for the degree of anaemia. A bone marrow aspirate, although very rarely per-

(a)

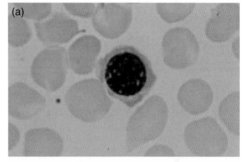

(b)

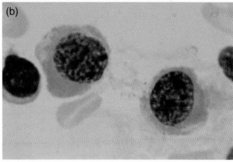

Figure 3.11 (a) Early polychromatic normoblast from the marrow of a healthy subject. (b) Early polychromatic megaloblasts from a patient with severe pernicious anaemia. These cells are larger and have a more delicate, sieve-like nucleus containing smaller particles of condensed chromatin than the early polychromatic normoblast.

formed, would show nuclear–cytoplasmic dyssynchrony and giant metamyelocytes (Figures 3.11–3.13). The destruction of defective erythroid cells in the

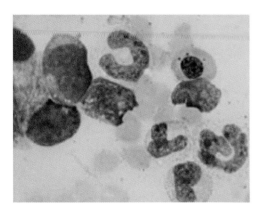

Figure 3.12 Two giant metamyelocytes near a normal-sized metamyelocyte in a marrow smear from a patient with untreated pernicious anaemia. There is also a megaloblast containing Howell–Jolly bodies (i.e. micronuclei).

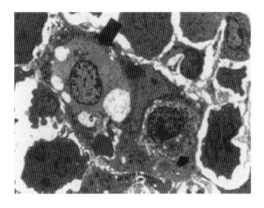

Figure 3.13 Electron micrograph of a bone marrow macrophage from a patient with severe pernicious anaemia. The cytoplasm of the macrophage contains two ingested megaloblasts (arrowed) at various stages of degradation.

marrow will result in a mild increase in bilirubin and lactate dehydrogenase (LDH) levels (see also Chapter 4).

Folic acid levels may be assayed in the serum and in the red cells themselves. However, the critical role of vitamin B12 in regenerating functional tetrahydrofolate means that low red cell folate levels may also be seen as a secondary effect in B12 deficiency. Moreover, although treating with folate supplementation when the primary defect is actually with B12 may temporarily ameliorate the haematological symptoms and signs, it will permit worsening of any B12-associated

neurological pathology. B12 levels should therefore be routinely tested alongside folic acid levels, and folate should never be supplemented alone where B12 and folate deficiency coexist.

Testing for B12 deficiency may not be as straightforward as a simple serum vitamin B12 assay. The great majority of assayed B12 in the serum is protein bound as part of 'haptocorrin', a form that is not functionally active; only B12 bound to the protein transcobalamin is physiologically available. Thus, any condition that affects the distribution of B12-binding proteins in the serum can affect the result of B12 assays. Pregnancy and the oral contraceptive pill, for example, can give falsely low B12 results, while some myeloproliferative disorders (which increase haptocorrin production) give falsely high readings. If in doubt, the substrates of the cobalamin-requiring enzymes can be assayed; both homocysteine and methylmalonic acid levels will be high in true B12 deficiency.

Finding the cause of deficiency is also important. A clear dietary history, consideration of tests for malabsorption, tissue transglutaminase antibodies (if coeliac disease is suspected as a cause of folate deficiency) and anti-intrinsic factor antibodies (to look for pernicious anaemia as a cause of B12 deficiency) should all be considered. The poor specificity of a finding of anti-gastric parietal cell antibodies means that testing is not advised in the diagnosis of pernicious anaemia.

Treatment

In all cases, the underlying cause must be treated where possible. Folic acid supplementation orally is generally sufficient to treat folic acid deficiency, though care must be taken to ensure that coincident B12 deficiency is not missed. Oral B12 supplements may help where there is simple dietary deficiency of B12 but clearly in pernicious anaemia, parenteral vitamin B12 administration by intramuscular injection is required and should continue lifelong.

Other causes of megaloblastosis

Conditions other than vitamin B12 and folate deficiency can cause megaloblastic erythropoiesis. Frequently, aberrations in the metabolism of vitamin B12 and folate are at the root of the megaloblastosis (consider the effects of methotrexate, which inhibits an enzyme critical for tetrahydrofolate production; or chronic nitrous oxide exposure, which can combine with the cobalt of cobalamin to inhibit its ability to function as an enzymatic cofactor), but any other drug or clinical condition that inhibits DNA synthesis will have a similar effect, as summarized in Box 3.6.

Box 3.0 **Vitamin B12-independent and folate-independent causes of macrocytosis with megaloblastic haematopoiesis**

Abnormalities of nucleic acid synthesis
- Drug therapy

   o Antipurines (mercaptopurine, azathioprine)
   o Antipyrimidines (fluorouracil, zidovudine)
   o Others (hydroxycarbamide)

- Orotic aciduria

Uncertain aetiology
- Myelodysplastic syndromes,[a] erythroleukaemia
- Some congenital dyserythropoietic anaemias

[a]Some patients show normoblastic erythropoiesis.

Normoblastic macrocytosis

Not all cases of macrocytic anaemia will be caused by megaloblastic changes in the marrow. Conditions in which macrocytosis is seen in the context of normoblastic erythropoiesis include alcohol excess (probably the most common cause of macrocytosis in the UK), liver dysfunction and hypothyroidism. The mechanisms underlying the macrocytosis in these cases are not always fully defined but all are characterized by abnormalities in lipid metabolism, which may be relevant. It is also possible for a marked expansion in erythroid output to produce a mild macrocytosis, as reticulocytes are slightly larger than more mature red cells. A summary of the causes of normoblastic macrocytosis is given in Box 3.7.

Box 3.7 Causes of vitamin B12- and folate-independent macrocytosis with normoblastic erythropoiesis

Normal neonates (physiological)
Chronic alcohol excess[a]
Myelodysplastic syndromes[a]
Chronic liver disease[a]
Hypothyroidism
Normal pregnancy
Therapy with anticonvulsant drugs[a]
Haemolytic anaemia
Hypoplastic and aplastic anaemia
Myeloma

[a]Some patients show B12- and folate-independent megaloblastic erythropoiesis.

Spurious elevations in the MCV may be seen in hyperglycaemia, thought to be a consequence of osmotic dysequilibrium between the red cells and the diluent used in preparing the cells for analysis.

Polycythaemia (erythrocytosis)

Just as perturbation of mechanisms controlling normal red cell production may result in anaemia, so dysregulation of these mechanisms may result in too many red cells being produced. The term 'polycythaemia' refers to an excess of red cells, such that the packed cell volume (also known as the haematocrit) of peripheral blood is consistently elevated (>0.52 in adult males and >0.48 in adult females). Polycythaemia may result either from an increase in the total volume of red cells in the circulation (true polycythaemia) or from a decrease in the total plasma volume (apparent or relative polycythaemia). These are discussed in more detail in Chapter 8, but a brief overview of true polycythaemia is given below.

True polycythaemia

An absolute increase in circulating red cells may arise from dysregulation of any of the mechanisms controlling normal red cell production. Thus, hypoxia secondary to chronic pulmonary disease or cyanotic heart disease will increase erythropoietin production, with a resultant stimulation of erythroid drive in the bone marrow. High-affinity haemoglobins, which fail to yield oxygen appropriately in the peripheral tissues, may also be responsible for an increased hypoxic signal and thus increased erythropoiesis. In normoxaemic conditions, inappropriate release of erythropoietin can occur in the context of renal tumours or polycystic kidney disease. Each of these cases will cause a true polycythaemia, but the ultimate cause in each case is extrinsic to the bone marrow: they are therefore termed 'secondary polycythaemias'. In each case, the serum epo level will be elevated.

Primary polycythaemia, also known as polycythaemia vera, arises from a defect in the haematopoietic system itself. It is characterized by the autonomous, epo-independent proliferation of erythroid precursors in the marrow. In the overwhelming majority of cases, this is caused by the acquisition of a mutation in the gene for JAK2, a protein tyrosine kinase that is critical for the downstream signalling through the epo receptor. Over 95% of patients with polycythaemia vera have the *JAK2* V617F mutation, which results in epo-independent red cell proliferation. A further mutation in exon 12 of the *JAK2* gene has also been described, with similar effects. In these conditions, negative feedback on the normal mechanisms for stimulating erythropoiesis will result in a low serum epo level.

The differential diagnosis of polycythaemia, and an approach to its management, are described in Chapter 8.

4

Haemolytic anaemias

LEARNING OBJECTIVES

After reading this chapter, you should be able to:

✔ define haemolysis and haemolytic anaemia

✔ understand the tests for recognizing haemolysis and the marrow response to it

✔ classify haemolytic anaemias into congenital and acquired types

✔ understand the difference between intravascular and extravascular haemolysis, and recognize the laboratory features of each

✔ describe the mode of inheritance, biochemical basis and clinical and laboratory features of hereditary spherocytosis

✔ understand the normal role of glucose-6-phosphate dehydrogenase and the pathogenesis and clinical characteristics of the haemolytic syndromes associated with its deficiency

✔ to appreciate that some disorders of globin function such as sickle cell disease are subtypes of haemolytic anaemia

✔ describe the role of autoantibodies in the development of haemolytic anaemias and know the types of disease with which they are associated

✔ recognize causes of non-immune acquired haemolytic anaemias.

Haemolysis is the shortening of the lifespan of a mature red blood cell. Small or moderate reductions in red cell survival need not produce an obvious clinical effect as increased red cell output from the marrow, stimulated by erythropoietin in response to hypoxaemia, will be sufficient to compensate for the accelerated red cell destruction. However, more marked reductions in red cell lifespan – say to 5–10 days, from the usual 120 days – will outstrip the capacity of the marrow to expand erythroid output and will result in *haemolytic anaemia*.

This compensatory increase in erythroid output requires an adequately functioning bone marrow and effective erythropoiesis. However, a suboptimal marrow response is seen when there are insufficient haematinics (iron, vitamin B12 or folate), when the red cell precursors are damaged, when the marrow is infiltrated by malignant cells or when there is ineffective

Haematology Lecture Notes, Eleventh Edition. Deborah Hay, Andrew King and Michael Desborough.
© 2023 John Wiley & Sons Ltd. Published 2023 by John Wiley & Sons Ltd.
Companion website: www.wiley.com/go/Hay/Haematology/11e

erythropoiesis, such as in thalassaemia. In each of these conditions, haemolysis will result in anaemia more readily.

In the majority of haemolytic anaemias, the red cell destruction is the result of phagocytosis by macrophages in the spleen, liver and bone marrow. This is termed *extravascular* haemolysis. By contrast, in *intravascular* haemolysis, the red cells are caused to rupture and release their haemoglobin (Hb) directly into the circulation. The intra- or extravascular site of red cell destruction can be determined by clinical laboratory investigations, and may give clues to the underlying aetiology of the haemolysis – in turn guiding effective treatment.

Clinical features of haemolysis

The haemolytic anaemias vary greatly in their clinical presentations. Some produce a mild, chronic, well-compensated haemolytic picture, while others manifest acutely with brisk haemolysis and a rapid drop in haemoglobin. As discussed in Chapter 3, this difference in the rate of drop of haemoglobin can have a major impact on the degree of clinical compromise that the patient experiences.

The different clinical presentations seen with different causes of haemolysis are discussed further in the following sections, but there are several clinical features common to all which should prompt the clinician to consider a diagnosis of haemolysis. First, pallor will be seen as a result of the low haemoglobin (Hb). Since there is accelerated red cell breakdown, the breakdown products of haemoglobin can accumulate (see Laboratory features, below), and the bilirubin may be sufficiently elevated to cause clinically detectable jaundice.

Splenomegaly may be present. In chronic haemolysis, this may reflect the spleen's role in extramedullary erythropoiesis when the capacity of the normal marrow cavities to support red cell production is exceeded, while in florid acute haemolytic anaemias it may reflect the volume of red cells being phagocytosed in the spleen. Long-term complications of chronic haemolysis include expansion of erythropoiesis in the marrow cavities, thinning of cortical bone, bone deformities (e.g. frontal and parietal bossing) and, very occasionally, pathological fractures. Pigment gallstones, composed of excess bilirubin, are seen commonly.

Laboratory evidence of haemolysis

Although clinical features may give a suggestion of the presence of haemolysis, laboratory testing will provide stronger data to support this. Both biochemical and haematological laboratory investigations can provide evidence of haemolysis. When red cells are destroyed, either in the circulation or by the macrophages of the spleen, liver or marrow, their haem group is converted first to biliverdin and then to bilirubin. Unconjugated bilirubin is insoluble and is transported to the liver bound to albumin; here it undergoes glucuronidation to facilitate its excretion. However, with increased red cell destruction, the glucuronidase can become saturated and unconjugated bilirubin will accumulate. Thus, haemolysis, whether intravascular or extravascular, will result in a rise in the unconjugated bilirubin concentration in the plasma.

Lactate dehydrogenase (LDH), one of the glycolytic pathway enzymes present in red cells, is also released as these cells are lysed. Breakdown of red cells intravascularly can result in very marked elevation of the serum LDH, while breaches in the red cell membrane caused by partial phagocytosis in extravascular haemolysis may also cause the serum LDH level to climb.

Some additional laboratory tests give an indication of the likely intravascular or extravascular nature of the haemolysis. When red cells are lysed intravascularly, free haemoglobin is released; this is bound by the protein haptoglobin, thereby limiting its potentially harmful oxidative effects. The haemoglobin-haptoglobin complex is taken up by hepatocytes and the complex is metabolized. The result is a low or even absent plasma haptoglobin. In severe intravascular haemolysis, when all available haptoglobin may be saturated with haemoglobin, free haem can bind to albumin to form methaemalbumin. This is also detectable biochemically, though this test is performed only infrequently. Unbound free haemoglobin can be detected in the plasma as well, and may pass through the renal glomeruli to give free haemoglobin in the urine; this is haemoglobinuria (note the difference from haematuria, which describes the presence of intact red cells in the urine). Haemoglobin may also be taken up by the renal tubular cells and converted to the iron storage complex haemosiderin. This can be detected with Perls' stain of spun deposits of urine, both in shed tubular cells and extracellularly.

Haematologically, all forms of haemolysis are expected to be characterized by evidence of increased erythroid drive, manifest through an increased reticulocyte count. The number of reticulocytes in the blood is expressed either as a percentage of the total number of red cells or as an absolute number per litre of blood; in normal adults, the percentage is in the range of 0.5–3.0% and the absolute count is 20–100 × 10^9/L. An increase in the absolute reticulocyte count is an indication of increased erythropoietic activity and, in general, the higher the count, the greater the rate of delivery of viable red cells to the circulation. The reticulocyte percentage may increase up to 50% or more when erythropoietic activity is intense, as in brisk haemolysis, though it should be noted that reticulocytosis is not a feature specific to haemolysis; it will be observed whenever there is increased erythroid drive, such as during the response to acute blood loss or following the replacement of vitamin B12, folic acid or iron in a setting of anaemia secondary to haematinic deficiency.

The slightly larger size of reticulocytes relative to mature red cells will lead to a small increase in the mean cell volume. As haemolysis will also increase the marrow's demand for folic acid, macrocytosis may also develop secondary to folate deficiency if this increased demand is not met by adequate intake (see also Chapter 3).

Any condition which limits a haemolysing patient's ability to mount a reticulocyte response will result in a precipitous fall in the Hb level (Box 4.1).

Box 4.1 Parvovirus in patients with haemolytic anaemias

Patients with haemolytic conditions are also at risk of episodes of pure red cell aplasia (see also Chapter 11). In this condition, which is typically the result of infection with parvovirus (also termed erythrovirus) B19, there is a complete or near complete failure of erythroid maturation. Parvovirus binds to the carbohydrate P-antigen on erythroid progenitor cell surfaces and exerts a directly cytotoxic effect. In patients with a normal red cell lifespan, the temporary cessation of erythroid maturation it causes may produce a dip in the haemoglobin level, but it is usually clinically insignificant from a haematological perspective. However, in haemolytic states, the combination of reticulocytopenia and a pre-existing shortened red cell lifespan can have a catastrophic effect on the Hb level. Affected patients may require urgent red cell transfusion.

The blood film is an essential investigation in efforts to understand the nature of a patient's haemolysis. Some features are consistent across all forms of haemolysis: the increased reticulocyte count can be detected visually on the film, since reticulocytes are both slightly larger and also have a different staining characteristic. These younger cells will contain more RNA than more mature red cells, and will therefore develop a more basophilic (blue) appearance on standard blood film staining. This variation in red cell staining is termed *polychromasia*.

The peripheral blood film in haemolysis will vary according to the underlying cause, and specific morphological features of different haemolytic anaemias are described in more detail in the following sections. However, generally, extravascular haemolysis is associated with spherocytosis on the peripheral blood film, because of the partial phagocytosis of red cells by the macrophages in the spleen, which distorts their surface area-to-volume ratio, while intravascular haemolysis is characterized by red cell fragmentation (schistocytes), as might be expected in the setting of direct trauma to red cells in the circulation.

In cases where examination of the bone marrow is undertaken, there will be evidence of increased erythropoiesis. A semiquantitative assessment of the degree of erythroid hyperplasia can be obtained by determining the myeloid:erythroid ratio in the bone marrow. This is defined as the ratio between the number of cells of the granulocyte series (including mature neutrophils) and the number of erythroblasts of all stages of maturation in bone marrow, with a normal ratio being approximately 3:1. Marrow samples with erythroid hyperplasia are also hypercellular, because of the replacement of fat cells by erythroblasts (Figure 4.1). In chronic haemolysis, haematopoietic tissue may extend beyond the confines of the normal red marrow-containing bones into marrow cavities that usually contain only fat, and extramedullary haematopoiesis may develop in the liver and spleen.

Again, these haematological features are not specific to haemolysis. Erythroid hyperplasia will also be seen after haemorrhage, in megaloblastic and sideroblastic anaemias, and in thalassaemia (where erythropoiesis is markedly ineffective; see Chapters 3 and 5), as well as in neoplastic conditions such as polycythaemia vera and erythroleukaemia.

The laboratory features of haemolysis are summarized in Table 4.1.

(a) (b)

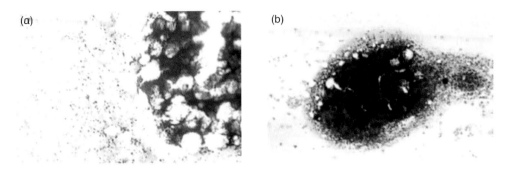

Figure 4.1 (a) A normocellular marrow fragment; about half its volume consists of haematopoietic cells (staining blue) and the remainder of unstained rounded fat cells. (b) A markedly hypercellular marrow fragment, as might be seen in the response to haemolysis; virtually all the fat cells are replaced by haematopoietic cells.

Table 4.1 Laboratory findings indicative of haemolysis.

	Extravascular haemolysis	Intravascular haemolysis
Hyperbilirubinaemia (unconjugated)	Present	Present
Reduced or absent serum haptoglobin	Unusual	Present
Haemoglobinuria, haemosiderinuria	Unusual	Present
Increased serum lactate dehydrogenase	Present	Present, often very high
Reticulocytosis	Present	Present
Blood film findings	Typically includes spherocytes	Typically includes red cell fragmentation

Classifying haemolytic anaemias and establishing a diagnosis

The laboratory and clinical features above describe general aspects of haemolytic states, but are not able to define the underlying cause of haemolysis – of which there are many. In thinking about the possible causes of haemolysis, a simple classification starts by dividing these initially into inherited and acquired causes. With the congenital causes, the underlying defect is typically intrinsic to the red cell itself, affecting the red cell membrane/cytoskeleton, its enzymes or its haemoglobin. Acquired causes, by contrast, are typically (but not exclusively) a result of defects outside the red cell, and can be divided into those with an immune basis and those which are non-immune.

This overview is summarized in Figure 4.2 and the individual conditions are outlined in the following sections.

Congenital haemolytic anaemias

Haemolysis resulting from defects of the red cell membrane and cytoskeleton

As the diameter of a normal red cell is similar to that of the smallest capillary lumen, it is essential for the red cell to be able to undergo significant deformations while traversing the circulation, while at the same time maintaining its structural integrity and

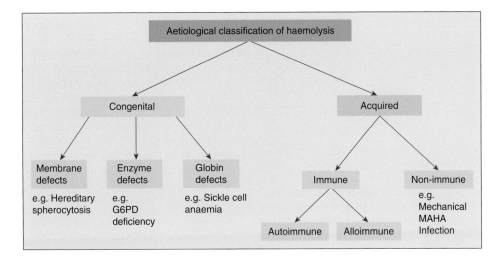

Figure 4.2 A classification of haemolytic anaemia by aetiology. G6PD, glucose-6-phosphate dehydrogenase; MAHA, microangiopathic haemolytic anaemia.

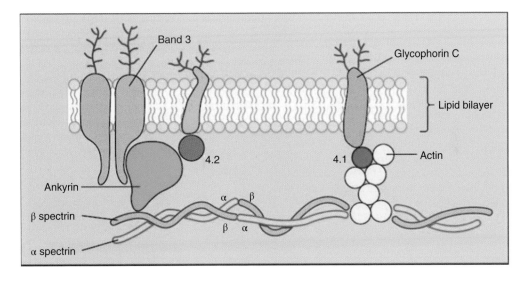

Figure 4.3 Schematic diagram of the red cell membrane cytoskeleton showing key proteins implicated in the pathophysiology of hereditary spherocytosis.

avoiding fragmentation. These contrasting requirements are accomplished through a flexible red cell cytoskeleton, which interacts with the red cell phospholipid membrane. Key components of the cytoskeleton include α and β spectrin, actin and protein 4.1, while connections linking the cytoskeleton to the overlying red cell phospholipid bilayer include band 3, Rh-associated glycoprotein and glycophorin C (Figure 4.3). Defects in any of these proteins can jeopardize the integrity of the red cell and shorten its lifespan.

Hereditary spherocytosis

The most common haemolytic anaemia resulting from a membrane defect is hereditary spherocytosis (HS), which affects 1 in 3000 people of northern European ancestry. At a genetic level, this disorder is heterogeneous, with mutations being seen in genes for several key proteins which provide vertical links between the red cell cytoskeleton and the cell membrane. Of these, mutations in spectrin, ankyrin and band 3 are the most common, with band 4.2 mutations also being frequently seen. The application of next-generation sequencing technology to previously undiagnosed kindreds has uncovered a range of additional genes implicated in this disorder, but in a minority of cases no molecular cause can be identified. Although the bulk of kindreds show autosomal dominant inheritance, autosomal recessive patterns have also been identified in some families.

The consequence of uncoupling the connections between the membrane and the cytoskeleton is a tendency to release bilayer lipids in the form of cytoskeleton-free vesicles. This leads to a loss of membrane surface area, with red cells adopting a spheroid rather than the normal biconcave shape. Repeated passage through the spleen aggravates this spherocytic change. Being less deformable than normal red cells, the passage of spherocytes through the splenic cords is hampered; the trapped cells are engulfed and destroyed by splenic macrophages, leading to a reduction in red cell survival by extravascular haemolysis.

As might be expected from a condition so heterogeneous at the molecular level, HS is highly variable in its clinical presentation. Around 20% of all patients with HS have mild disease with well-compensated haemolysis. These patients will have a near normal haemoglobin maintained by a higher than normal reticulocyte count, and will have only mild spherocytosis and mild splenomegaly. Indeed, such patients may not even present to medical attention until they develop complications of chronic haemolysis in adulthood (e.g. gallstones). The majority of patients have moderate disease characterized by a Hb concentration of 80–110 g/L, while a small percentage have severe disease requiring intermittent or even regular transfusions.

Complications of the chronic haemolysis in HS include the development of pigment gallstones (sometimes associated with biliary obstruction). Aplastic crises may occur secondary to parvovirus B19 infection and it should be noted than many otherwise trivial intercurrent infections can lead to episodes of increased haemolysis, sometimes requiring transfusion. Megaloblastic anaemia resulting from folate deficiency is also occasionally found, as in other chronic haemolytic disorders. This results from an increased requirement for folate by the hyperactive bone marrow, and is especially found when the diet is inadequate.

Diagnosis and management

The cardinal clinical features are a family history, mild jaundice, pallor and splenomegaly, but clearly these may not distinguish HS from other forms of inherited haemolytic anaemia. Laboratory findings include the general features of haemolysis (anaemia, reticulocytosis and elevated plasma bilirubin), but also the presence of spherocytes on the peripheral blood film (Figure 4.4). While spherocytes are also typically seen in patients with autoimmune haemolytic anaemia, discussed below, their presence in the context of a positive family history and a negative direct antiglobulin test will strongly suggest HS – and, indeed, no further diagnostic testing may be required in such patients.

Where more definitive evidence for the diagnosis is needed, the eosin-5-maleamide (EMA) binding test may be used. EMA is a fluorescent dye that binds the transmembrane protein band 3 on the red cell surface. The extent of binding can be gauged by a flow cytometric analysis of a fluorescent signal from the cell surface (see Chapter 7 for further discussion of flow cytometry). HS, and other membrane disorders that result in disruption of the red cell cytoskeleton and its linkage to the phospholipid bilayer, will result in decreased EMA binding and a reduced fluorescent signal. An appreciation of which protein is affected may not be required for the clinical care of the patient, but if it is, or if other tests have yielded borderline results, the red cell membrane proteins may also be subject to electrophoresis on a denaturing

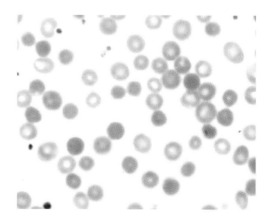

Figure 4.4 A blood film from a patient with hereditary spherocytosis showing many spherocytes. These are the smaller, more densely staining cells which lack the usual area of central pallor.

polyacrylamide gel. Increasingly, next-generation sequencing is used as an alternative diagnostic test, though the great variation in mutations from family to family with HS means this is not always a simple diagnostic strategy.

The treatment of HS should be tailored to the severity of the individual case. All patients should receive folic acid supplementation, in light of their increased rate of erythropoiesis. Children with severe disease are likely to require splenectomy; this should also be considered for those with moderately severe disease. As well as markedly reducing haemolysis and lengthening the red cell lifespan, this will reduce the likelihood of developing many long-term complications. However, splenectomy will increase the risk of significant infection, particularly from encapsulated organisms such as *Neisseria meningitidis* and *Streptococcus pneumoniae*. This risk is especially marked in children under the age of 5, and splenectomy is therefore typically delayed until the child is 5–10 years old. Pre-splenectomy preparation should include the administration of pneumococcal and meningococcal vaccines and *Haemophilus influenzae* type b vaccine; although the data to support antibiotic prophylaxis with penicillin V are limited, many centres advise this lifelong post-splenectomy, in an attempt to prevent the development of serious infection by encapsulated organisms. There is also evidence that splenectomy increases the risk of venous thromboembolic disease (see also Chapter 14).

Hereditary elliptocytosis and hereditary pyropoikilocytosis

Hereditary elliptocytosis (HE) is seen especially in regions where malaria is endemic. As with HS, it is an inherited haemolytic disorder caused by red cell cytoskeleton defects, and is heterogeneous at both a molecular and clinical level. The majority of kindreds have defects in α spectrin, though other components of the red cell cytoskeleton may be affected. While most patients are clinically asymptomatic, some will have a chronic symptomatic haemolytic anaemia. All show the very characteristic red cell shape on peripheral blood films (Figure 4.5).

Where there is severe disturbance of the multimerization of spectrin, patients usually have a severe haemolytic anaemia from infancy, with bizarre peripheral blood morphology, including microspherocytes and poikilocytes. Such patients are described as having hereditary pyropoikilocytosis; molecular analysis shows that this is the homozygous or compound heterozygous state for the mutations that cause HE.

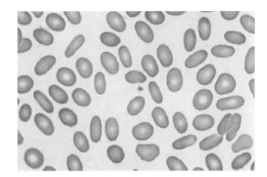

Figure 4.5 A blood film from a patient with hereditary elliptocytosis showing a high proportion of elliptical red cells.

Haemolysis caused by abnormalities of red cell enzymes

Haemolytic anaemias may also result from congenital abnormalities of the enzymes required for energy transfer in glucose metabolism. The red cell needs a continuous supply of energy for the maintenance of membrane flexibility and cell shape, the regulation of sodium and potassium pumps, and the maintenance of Hb in the reduced ferrous form. As mature red cells lack mitochondria, there is a reliance on the anaerobic glycolytic pathway for glucose metabolism and ATP generation.

There is also an alternative direct oxidative pathway for glucose metabolism, the pentose-phosphate shunt, in which glucose-6-phosphate is directly oxidized, eventually leading to the production of metabolites that can rejoin the anaerobic glycolytic pathway. Although this shunt does not yield ATP directly, it is capable of reducing NADP+ to NADPH, which in turn can be oxidized to maintain reduced glutathione (GSH). The significance of the pentose-phosphate shunt is therefore its ability to provide a pool of 'reducing activity' in the form of GSH that can be used to keep the sulfhydryl groups of haemoglobin, red cell enzymes and membrane proteins in their functional reduced forms (Figure 4.6).

Glucose-6-phosphate dehydrogenase deficiency

Deficiency of glucose-6-phosphate dehydrogenase (G6PD), the first enzyme of the pentose-phosphate shunt, will prevent the normal generation of NADPH, with subsequent erythrocyte sensitivity to oxidative stress. The molecular basis of G6PD deficiency is

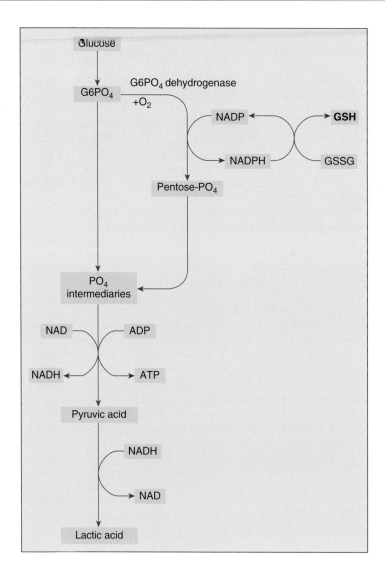

Figure 4.6 A schematic diagram of the pathway of glucose metabolism in the red cell, to show the important role of G6PD. Decreased activity of the enzyme leads to a deficiency of the reducing compounds NADPH and glutathione (GSH). NAD, nicotinamide adenine dinucleotide; NADH, reduced nicotinamide adenine dinucleotide; NADP, nicotinamide adenine dinucleotide phosphate; GSH, Glutathione (reduced form); GSSG, glutathione disulphide (oxidised form).

highly variable, with various point mutations in the G6PD gene on the X chromosome resulting in altered enzyme activity and kinetics. The normal G6PD enzyme is designated type B and is the prevalent form worldwide; G6PD type A is a normal variant found in approximately 20% of healthy individuals of African ancestry. Defective forms of G6PD include the A– African variant, in which the enzyme activity is reduced to approximately one-tenth of its normal function, and the Mediterranean variant in which the enzyme activity is even more markedly limited, at 1–3% of normal. Together, these two mutations account for >95% of all cases of G6PD deficiency.

The gene for G6PD is found on the X chromosome, and affected individuals are male (homozygous women are affected as well but are unusual; skewed lionization may also give reduced enzyme activity in some heterozygous women). It has been estimated that as many as 400 million people worldwide are affected, with the prevalence being high in areas where malaria is endemic. It has been shown that the deficiency affords some protection against *Plasmodium falciparum* malaria, with heterozygous females infected with malaria having lower parasitaemia than women without G6PD deficiency. This selective pressure has led to deficiency of the enzyme in about 20% of individuals of west and central African origin, and is also found to a varying extent in southern Europe, the Middle East, India, Thailand and southern China. It is rare in people of northern European ethnicity.

Since G6PD has a critical role in maintaining the pool of reducing power in the erythrocyte, patients with low levels of the enzyme are poorly protected against oxidative challenge. In these patients, exposure to some medications and even some foods (broad beans are the best known example) can result in marked oxidative damage to the red cell. When the red cell is exposed to these oxidants, haemoglobin is oxidized to form methaemoglobin and denatured haemoglobin then precipitates, forming inclusions in the red cell (termed Heinz bodies and detected by supravital staining, as in Figure 4.7).

Heinz bodies, and the portion of the red cell membrane to which they become attached, are removed by splenic macrophages as the red cells pass through the spleen; the resulting inclusion-free cells display unstained areas at their periphery ('bite' cells, seen in Figure 4.8). Red cells with oxidative membrane damage are removed extravascularly by the spleen, though acute responses to a severe oxidative challenge may also provoke intravascular haemolysis.

Oxidant drugs that may bring about this type of haemolytic anaemia include antimalarials (e.g. primaquine), sulfonamides, quinolones, nitrofurantoin, aspirin (in high doses), some non-steroidal anti-inflammatories, rasburicase and vitamin K analogues.

A number of screening tests and assays for detecting G6PD deficiency are available. These are based on assessing the production of NADPH by red cells in the presence of an excess of glucose-6-phosphate. The NADPH is detected spectrophotometrically, or by its ability to reduce nitroblue tetrazolium (NBT) in the presence of an electron transfer agent, or by its fluorescence in ultraviolet light.

A variety of clinical syndromes may be associated with G6PD variants that have reduced enzyme activity.

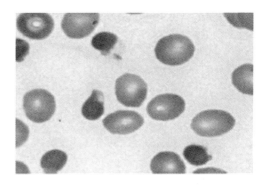

Figure 4.8 'Bite' cells in the blood film of a patient with G6PD deficiency who had received primaquine. These red cells are irregular in shape, abnormally dense and show a poorly staining area just beneath part of the cell membrane (MGG stain).

The most common of these is episodic acute haemolysis. For most of the time, patients with the two common G6PD variants (A- and Mediterranean types) are well and have normal Hb concentrations with only a slight shortening of the red cell lifespan. Episodes of haemolytic anaemia develop during infections or following exposure to oxidant drugs and chemicals. Haemolysis typically begins 1–3 days following exposure to the oxidative stressor, with anaemia being maximal about 7–10 days after exposure. The extent of the fall in Hb concentration is partly dependent on the amount and nature of the drug being given, and partly on the extent of the reduction of enzyme activity. During this time, the patient may report dark urine because of haemoglobinuria. A subtype of acute haemolysis is favism, a syndrome in which an acute haemolytic anaemia occurs after the ingestion of the broad (fava) bean (*Vicia fava*) in individuals with a deficiency of G6PD (commonly of the Mediterranean type). Favism usually affects children; severe anaemia develops rapidly and is often accompanied by haemoglobinuria. Fava beans contain two β-glycosides, vicine and convicine, which generate free radicals and consequently oxidize GSH and other red cell constituents.

Although the majority of patients with G6PD deficiency have episodic haemolytic episodes, some patients with severe enzyme defects have a more chronic haemolytic picture, with oxidative exacerbations. In these patients, the chronic haemolysis is principally extravascular.

A further possible presentation of G6PD deficiency is in infancy, with hyperbilirubinaemia. A combination of oxidative damage to red cells alongside immaturity of the bilirubin-conjugating system can lead

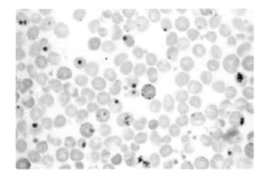

Figure 4.7 Membrane-bound Heinz bodies consisting of denatured haemoglobin (supravital staining with methyl violet).

to hyperbilirubinaemia, sometimes necessitating exchange transfusion. Affected individuals recover completely after the neonatal period, but may develop episodic acute haemolysis during later life.

Treatment of G6PD deficiency

Treatment focuses on the avoidance of oxidative precipitants to haemolysis. In many cases, haemolysis is self-limiting; in patients with the A– variant, for example, after about 10 days the Hb concentration starts to climb and may reach normal levels, even with continuation of the offending oxidant drug. This is because in these patients, only the older red cells have sufficiently low G6PD levels to be affected; as the reticulocyte count rises, so the effect of exposure to the oxidant is diminished. For patients with the Mediterranean variant, in whom the average enzyme activity is lower, haemolytic episodes may not be self-limiting, and packed red cell transfusion may be required in cases of severe haemolysis.

Other red cell enzyme deficiencies causing haemolysis: pyruvate kinase deficiency

G6PD is not the only enzyme deficiency that can result in haemolysis. Pyruvate kinase deficiency is another relatively common example, affecting individuals of all ethnic groups. Pyruvate kinase is one of the key enzymes of the glycolytic pathway, and two isoforms are encoded by two separate genes. *PKLR* encodes isoforms generated in the red cell and liver, while *PKM* is a muscle-specific isoform. Mutations causing clinical haemolytic anaemia are therefore seen in the *PKLR* gene. The exact mechanism by which defects in pyruvate kinase lead to haemolysis remains unclear.

At a molecular level it is a highly heterogeneous condition, with most affected patients being compound heterozygotes. This heterogeneity is reflected in the clinical presentation, but there is usually a chronic haemolytic anaemia and severely affected patients may benefit from splenectomy. Reaching a formal diagnosis may be challenging, since blood film findings are often rather non-specific; however, biochemical estimation of PK activity can be performed, and genetic sequencing of the PKLR gene is now routinely undertaken in patients with a long-standing 'non-spherocytic' haemolytic anaemia.

Although the treatment for pyruvate kinase deficiency remains essentially supportive, newer targeted therapies are under evaluation. Mitapivat is a small molecule allosteric activator of the red cell isoform of pyruvate kinase, which has been shown to enhance the activity of both the wild-type enzyme and several mutated forms. Early studies suggest it can deliver significant and sustainable prolongation in red cell survival and better haemoglobin levels in patients with pyruvate kinase deficiency.

Haemolysis resulting from haemoglobin defects

The third category of congenital haemolytic anaemias relates to defects in the structure of haemoglobin. These conditions are summarized as part of the classification of haemolytic anaemias, but are discussed in more detail in Chapter 5. Briefly, structural variants of the globin chains may affect the lifespan of the red cell, with sickle cell anaemia being the best-described example. A tendency of the HbS variant to polymerize under conditions of low oxygen tension leads to distortion of the erythrocyte into the well-recognized sickle shape. The distorted cells are subject to both intra- and extravascular haemolysis.

Acquired haemolytic anaemias

In the acquired haemolytic anaemias, red cells are destroyed either by immunological or by non-immunological mechanisms.

Immune haemolytic anaemias

In these conditions, antigens on the surface of red cells react with antibodies, sometimes with complement activation. IgG-coated red cells interact with the Fc receptors on macrophages in the spleen, and are then either completely or partially phagocytosed. When the phagocytosis is partial, the damaged cell will return to the circulation as a spherocyte. Red cells that are also coated with the activated complement component C3 may interact with C3 receptors on macrophages and are usually completely phagocytosed. In most instances where complement is activated, the cascade sequence proceeds only as far as C3 deposition on the cell surface. In a few instances, activation of complement proceeds further and permits deposition of the membrane attack complex

(C5–C9) with resultant breach of the cell membrane and intravascular haemolysis.

The immune haemolytic anaemias may be caused by autoantibodies – that is, antibodies formed against one or more antigenic constituents of the individual's own tissues. These include autoimmune haemolytic anaemia (AIHA) and some drug-related haemolytic anaemias. However, it is also possible to develop alloimmune haemolytic anaemia, consequent on the production of antibodies against red cells from another individual, as in haemolytic transfusion reactions and haemolytic disease of the newborn (see Chapter 15). A further mechanism by which immune dysregulation can result in haemolysis is found in the rare condition paroxysmal nocturnal haemoglobinuria (PNH), which arises when an acquired defect in the red cell membrane leads to complement-mediated haemolysis (Box 4.2).

Autoimmune haemolytic anaemias

A classification of the autoimmune haemolytic anaemias (AIHA) is given in Box 4.3. The temperature dependence of the autoantibody's binding affinity for its red cell surface antigen will determine the clinical picture. 'Warm' autoantibodies react best with the red

---

Box 4.2

Paroxysmal nocturnal haemoglobinuria

This rare clonal disorder arises as a consequence of somatic mutation of the *PIG-A* gene in a multipotent haematopoietic stem cell. The product of the *PIG-A* gene is critical for forming the glycosylphosphatidyl-inositol (GPI) anchor, which links many membrane proteins to the phospholipid bilayer. Among the many GPI-anchored proteins are CD55 and CD59, also known as decay-accelerating factor and the membrane inhibitor of reactive lysis. These proteins are regulators of the complement pathway. Consequently, cells that lack the GPI anchor have reduced or absent CD55 and CD59 on their cell membranes, and are extremely sensitive to complement-mediated intravascular haemolysis.

The haemolysis of paroxysmal nocturnal haemoglobinuria (PNH) is generally chronic, although there may be acute exacerbations. Thrombosis is another clinical feature of PNH; while the mechanisms underlying it are not fully understood, it is known that some components of the fibrinolytic pathway are GPI linked, and free haemoglobin released in intravascular haemolysis may also have an activating effect on vascular endothelial cells.

The diagnosis is usually based on flow cytometry for the key GPI-anchored proteins CD55 and CD59. Newer techniques to diagnose PNH include FLAER (fluorescent labelled aerolysin), in which a bacterially derived aerolysin binds to the GPI anchor itself; thus, the absence of fluorescence due to FLAER in a population of myeloid cells will indicate the presence of a PNH clone. Treatment may be supportive (folic acid and iron supplementation, anticoagulation where needed), with treatments targeting the underlying pathophysiology such as eculizumab, a monoclonal antibody against the C5 component of complement, being available.

Paroxysmal cold haemoglobinuria

This rare disease, seen most commonly in children, is caused by an IgG antibody with anti-P specificity (P is a glycolipid red cell antigen). The antibody, called the Donath–Landsteiner antibody, is capable of binding complement and has a particular thermal profile of activity. The antibody and early complement components bind to red cells at cool temperatures but lysis occurs only on warming to 37 °C. A rapid screening test therefore consists of incubating the patient's red cells and serum at 4 °C and then warming the mixture to 37 °C (the Donath–Landsteiner test). As might be predicted, patients experience acute episodes of marked haemoglobinuria caused by severe intravascular haemolysis when exposed to the cold. An acute transient form associated with a viral infection (e.g. influenza, mumps, Epstein–Barr virus) affects children. The chronic form is usually seen in adults and is associated with syphilis. Idiopathic chronic PCH is rare.

Drug-induced haemolytic anaemia

There are several mechanisms by which drugs can induce a haemolytic anaemia. In some cases, the drug acts as a hapten and binds to red cell membrane proteins, inducing antibody formation. Penicillins and cephalosporins, especially in high doses, have been implicated in this form of haemolytic anaemia. Alpha methyldopa is another drug well known to produce haemolytic anaemia in some patients, through the interaction of autoantibodies with the red cell surface, even in the absence of the drug – a mechanism clearly distinct from the hapten mechanism or immune complex effect. Treatment in each case focuses on the withdrawal of the offending drug. As with other causes of immune haemolysis, transfusion is avoided where possible.

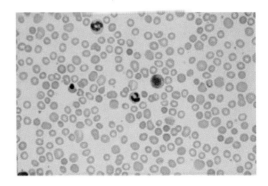

Figure 4.9 Blood film from a patient with idiopathic autoimmune haemolytic anaemia (AIHA) (warm-reactive antibody) showing prominent spherocytosis and polychromasia. A nucleated red blood cell is also visible on the left of the image.

cell antigen at 37 °C and are usually of IgG subtype. 'Cold' antibodies react best at temperatures below 32 °C (usually below 15 °C) and are usually of IgM subtype. As IgM is pentameric, these autoantibodies are capable of agglutinating red cells.

Warm AIHA

In idiopathic warm AIHA, haemolysis dominates the clinical picture and no evidence can be found of any other disease. In secondary AIHA, the haemolysis is associated with a primary disease such as chronic lymphocytic leukaemia or systemic lupus erythematosus (SLE). Some 50–70% of 'warm' autoantibodies show specificity for the Rh antigen system (see Chapter 15) and some of the remainder for other blood group antigen systems. The pathological mechanism by which these antibodies arise is unclear.

The antibody-coated red cells undergo partial or complete phagocytosis in the spleen and by the Kupffer cells of the liver. There may be partial activation of the complement cascade in addition, although completion to the membrane attack complex of complement is rare – a likely consequence of the activity of the complement regulatory proteins, factors I and H.

The clinical presentation of warm AIHA is highly variable but, unlike cold AIHA, it is unrelated to ambient temperature. Patients are usually over the age of 50. Some patients with florid haemolysis are very ill with an acute onset of severe anaemia accompanied by a brisk reticulocytosis; others have few or no symptoms and a mild chronic anaemia or even a compensated haemolytic state. Mild jaundice is common and splenomegaly may be found.

Haematological findings include anaemia, spherocytosis (Figure 4.9), reticulocytosis, occasional nucleated red cells in the peripheral blood and sometimes a neutrophil leucocytosis. However, the critical diagnostic investigation is the direct antiglobulin test (also known as the direct Coombs' test) (Figure 4.10).

In the direct antiglobulin test (DAT), washed red cells from the patient are incubated with an anti-human globulin. This globulin is able to bind to antibodies on the red cell surface. Being divalent, the antihuman globulin can bind IgG from two red cells, and is thus able to agglutinate cells that are coated with antibody. Such agglutination of red cells can be detected visually, and constitutes a positive DAT result. Cells that are not coated with IgG will remain unagglutinated, giving a negative DAT. The test can also be made specific for individual subtypes of IgG and for complement components that may be found on the red cell surface in AIHA. It should be noted, however, that a positive DAT result does not always imply active haemolysis; studies of healthy blood donors suggest that up to 1 in 10 000 of the population will have a positive test without haematological consequences.

In most patients, the haemolysis can be limited by treatment with prednisolone, which is initially given in high doses. If there is no response to steroids, or if the reduction in haemolysis is not maintained when the dose of steroids is lowered, alternative immunosuppressive therapy should be considered. The anti-CD20 monoclonal antibody rituximab, as well as immunosuppressants such as azathioprine, mycophenylate or cyclophosphamide, may be beneficial in reducing autoantibody production. Rarely, splenectomy may be needed. In patients with severe

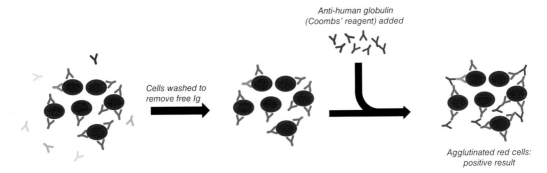

*Anti-human globulin
(Coombs' reagent) added*

*Cells washed to
remove free Ig*

*Agglutinated red cells:
positive result*

Figure 4.10 The direct antiglobulin test, also known as the direct Coombs' test, detects immunoglobulin bound to the red cell surface using an anti-human globulin. In this test, a sample of blood is taken from a patient with suspected autoimmune haemolytic anaemia. In this condition, the red cells are coated with an auto-antibody with a specificity for a red cell antigen. The cells are washed to remove any free immunoglobulin (Ig), and an anti-human globulin (antibody with specificity for the Fc portion of the human immunoglobulin) is added. This is the Coombs' reagent. In autoimmune haemolytic anaemia, this reagent is expected to cause agglutination of the red cells (a positive result). When performed on a sample in which the red cells are *not* bound by an autoantibody (i.e. patient without autoimmune haemolysis), the Coombs' reagent cannot cause red cell agglutination, and the test is negative.

anaemia and circulatory compromise, the least incompatible ABO- and Rh-matched blood should be transfused. However, transfusion is avoided wherever possible in AIHA, as even transfused cells can become coated with antibody and will have a relatively short half-life.

Cold autoimmune haemolysis

Since 'cold' IgM autoantibodies react with red cells only at temperatures below ~32 °C, they typically bind to the red cell surface in the cooler superficial blood vessels of the peripheries. Their pentameric structure permits direct agglutination of red cells coated with antibody; they are therefore sometimes termed *cold agglutinins*. This is readily seen in blood films made at room temperature (Figure 4.11).

Symptoms resulting from cold AIHA are worse during cold weather. Exposure to cold provokes acrocyanosis (coldness, purplish discoloration and numbness of fingers, toes, ear lobes and nose), caused by the formation of agglutinates of red cells in the vessels of the skin. The direct activation of the complement system by the IgM antibodies on the red cell surface leads to red cell lysis and, consequently, to haemoglobinaemia and haemoglobinuria.

A DAT will reveal that complement proteins are bound to the red cell surface, though the cold antibody itself frequently dissociates from the red cells during the washing phase of the test and may not be detected.

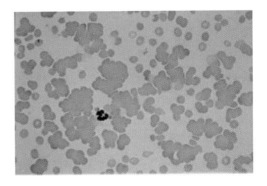

Figure 4.11 Numerous red cell agglutinates on a blood film from a patient with idiopathic cold haemagglutinin disease (CHAD).

The cold agglutinin in chronic idiopathic cold haemagglutinin disease (CHAD) is a *monoclonal* IgM antibody, normally with anti-I specificity (I and i are the names given to carbohydrate antigens on the surface of red cells; adult red cells contain more I than i determinants; see Chapter 15). The anti-I titre at 4 °C may be as high as 1 : 2000–500 000 (normal, 1 : 10–40). In all cases, it is important to look for the B-cell clone which is producing the monotypic IgM antibody; low-grade lymphoproliferative diseases should be sought by peripheral blood flow cytometry (see Chapter 7), but further investigation may also be required.

Chronic idiopathic CHAD is managed initially simply by keeping the patient warm. However, some patients remain symptomatic and treatment is required. Unlike warm AIHA, glucocorticoids and splenectomy tend to be of limited use. Treatment with rituximab may be effective. More recently, a monoclonal antibody targeted to the C1s component of complement, sutilimimab, has been found to be useful in early-stage trials, highlighting the importance of haemolysis of complement-opsonised red cells in the pathophysiology of this disorder.

Chronic idiopathic cold haemagglutinin disease has also been termed *primary* cold haemagglutinin disease, to separate it from secondary causes of cold haemolysis. In this latter category are infections and non-haematological malignancies which can induce cold immune haemolysis. Patients with *Mycoplasma* pneumonia or infectious mononucleosis, for example, develop acute self-limiting cold haemolytic anaemia, with production of polyclonal IgM antibodies of anti-I or anti-i specificity, respectively. Management here is typically supportive.

Other causes of haemolytic anaemia with an immune element to their pathogenesis include PNH, paroxysmal cold haemoglobinuria and some drug-related haemolytic anaemias (see Box 4.2).

Non-immune haemolytic anaemias

Mechanical damage to red cells

Several of the mechanical causes of acquired non-immune haemolytic anaemia are summarized in Box 4.4 (Figures 4.12–4.14). Red cells are mechanically damaged when they impact upon abnormal surfaces such as cardiac valve prostheses in valve-associated haemolysis, or activated vascular endothelium in the microangiopathic haemolytic anaemias. March haemoglobinuria is the result of intravascular haemolysis occurring after repeated red cell trauma in the small vessels of the feet, sometimes seen in marathon runners or training army cadets. In disseminated intravascular coagulation (see Chapter 13), inappropriate activation of the coagulation cascade produces fibrin strands which are thought to cause mechanical destruction of red cells. Such damage usually results in the presence of red cell fragments in the blood film and, because the red cells are damaged intravascularly, there may also be haemoglobinaemia, haemoglobinuria and an undetectable plasma haptoglobin.

> **Box 4.4 Causes of acquired non-immune haemolytic anaemias**
>
> - Mechanical trauma to red cells
>   - Abnormalities in the heart and large blood vessels, e.g. aortic valve prostheses (see Figure 4.12), severe aortic valve disease
>   - Microangiopathic haemolytic anaemia, e.g. haemolytic uraemic syndrome, thrombotic thrombocytopenic purpura, metastatic malignancy, accelerated hypertension, disseminated intravascular coagulation
>   - March haemoglobinuria
> - Burns
> - Infections: *Clostridium perfringens (welchii)*, malaria (see Figures 4.13 and 4.14), bartonellosis
> - Drugs,[a] chemicals and venoms: oxidant drugs and chemicals, acute lead poisoning, copper toxicity, venoms of certain spiders and snakes
> - Hypersplenism
>
> [a]Some drugs cause haemolysis by immune mechanisms.

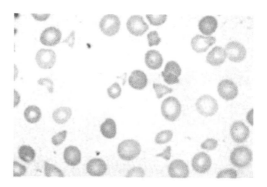

Figure 4.12 Fragmented red cells in the blood film of a patient with a malfunctioning aortic valve prosthesis.

Non-immune haemolytic anaemia resulting from drugs

While immune mechanisms of drug-induced haemolysis are well described, there are also non-immune mechanisms by which the red cell lifespan may be shortened. Chemicals such as benzene, toluene and saponin, which are fat solvents, act on the red cell membrane directly and disrupt its lipid components, inducing haemolysis. In addition, certain

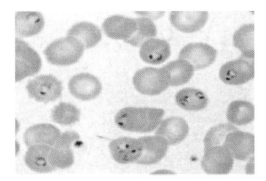

Figure 4.13 Blood film from a patient with *Plasmodium falciparum* malaria showing several parasitized red cells. Red cells heavily parasitized with malaria may be subject to intravascular lysis.

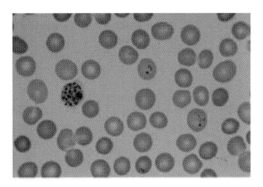

Figure 4.14 Blood film from a patient with *Plasmodium vivax* malaria showing two parasitized red cells, each containing a single parasite (ring form or early trophozoite and an amoeboid late trophozoite). Another red cell contains a schizont. Some of the parasitized cells are slightly enlarged.

drugs such as primaquine, the sulfonamides and phenacetin, which oxidize and denature Hb and other cell components in people with a deficiency of G6PD, can, if given in a large enough dose, also affect normal red cells. For example, the two oxidant drugs dapsone and sulfasalazine can cause haemolysis in healthy individuals when given in conventional doses.

Hypersplenism

Hypersplenism describes the reduction in the lifespan of red cells, granulocytes and platelets that may be found in patients with splenomegaly from any cause. The cytopenias found in patients with enlarged spleens are also partly caused by increased pooling of blood cells within the spleen and an increased plasma volume; the magnitude of both these effects is proportional to spleen size. In some haematological diseases in which anaemia is caused by a congenital or acquired defect of the red cell or impaired red cell formation, hypersplenism may have a role in worsening the anaemia, and splenectomy may be needed to address the effect.

5

Disorders of globin synthesis

LEARNING OBJECTIVES

After reading this chapter, you should be able to:

✔ describe the normal structure and function of haemoglobin

✔ recognize how the globin components of haemoglobin change during development

✔ understand the mechanisms by which the thalassaemias arise

✔ recognize the clinical presentations and complications of thalassaemia

✔ appreciate the contribution of haemolysis and ineffective erythropoiesis to the pathophysiology of thalassaemia

✔ describe the pathophysiology, presentation and complications of sickle cell anaemia

✔ understand the role of haemoglobin electrophoresis and high-performance liquid chromatography in the investigation of globin disorders

✔ appreciate that many other haemoglobin variants are associated with disease.

Disorders affecting the production of the globin chains which make up the haemoglobin molecule are among the most common genetic disorders in the world, and are responsible for a significant burden of morbidity and mortality. In order to understand attempts to treat and counsel affected patients accurately, we need to understand the normal structure and function of haemoglobin; these are reviewed briefly in the first part of this chapter. We then move on to an introduction to quantitative and qualitative disorders affecting haemoglobin production – the haemoglobinopathies.

Normal structure and function of haemoglobin

Haemoglobin is critical to the normal function of the red cell, the fundamental role of which is the transport of oxygen from the lungs to the tissues. The normal haemoglobin molecule comprises two 'α-like' globin polypeptide chains and two 'β-like' globin chains; each globin molecule is associated with a haem group, which comprises a porphyrin ring with iron in its ferrous form at the centre. It is to the iron in this haem group that oxygen binds.

In shifting between the oxygen unbound and bound states, the haemoglobin molecule undergoes conformational change, which enhances its affinity for the binding of subsequent molecules of oxygen. The physiological consequence of this is haemoglobin's sigmoidal oxygen binding curve, which enables it to load oxygen effectively in situations of high oxygen tension, yet also to release it effectively in the relatively low oxygen tension of the peripheral tissues.

In addition, several other ligands can allosterically influence the binding of oxygen to the haem groups. A by-product of glucose metabolism in the cell, 2,3-diphosphoglycerate (2,3-DPG), can bind to the globin chains and decrease the affinity of haemoglobin for oxygen, thus shifting the oxygen dissociation curve to the right. The effect is to facilitate the release of oxygen in a manner which is linked to the metabolic activity of the tissues. Likewise, a fall in the pH in the peripheral tissues or an increase in the CO_2 concentration (the Bohr effect) has similar consequences, such that the release of oxygen from the haemoglobin molecule to the tissues can be enhanced in the setting of increased metabolic demand (Figure 5.1).

The globin chain composition of haemoglobin can also influence its oxygen affinity. Although all normal haemoglobins consist of two pairs of distinct globin polypeptides, the precise nature of these globin chains changes during intrauterine and postnatal life. The α-like chains are encoded on chromosome 16 and their genes are arranged in the order in which they are expressed during development: the embryonic ζ globin gene first, followed by the adult α globin genes. The β-like globins are encoded on chromosome 11 and again are found in the order of their expression: the embryonic ε gene, followed by the fetal γ globin and the adult β globin gene. Thus, the complete haemoglobin molecule varies in its composition during development: Hb Gower ($\zeta_2\varepsilon_2$ and $\alpha_2\varepsilon_2$) and Hb

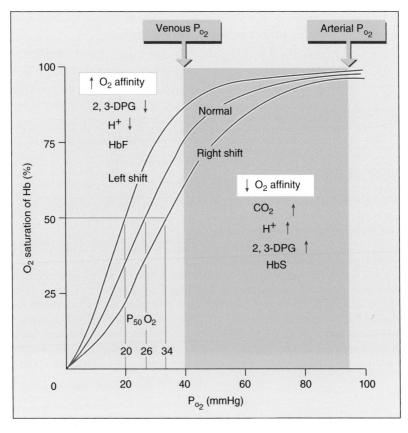

Figure 5.1 Oxygen–haemoglobin dissociation curves. 2,3-DPG, 2,3-diphosphoglycerate; HbS, sickle haemoglobin; HbF, fetal haemoglobin.

Portland ($\zeta_2\gamma_2$) are the earliest forms seen, followed by fetal haemoglobin HbF ($\alpha_2\gamma_2$), which persists for several months postnatally but contributes only a very small percentage of the normal adult complement of haemoglobins. The major adult haemoglobin is HbA ($\alpha_2\beta_2$), with a much smaller contribution from HbA2 ($\alpha_2\delta_2$, usually 1.5–3.5% of adult haemoglobins). The fetal haemoglobin HbF has a higher oxygen affinity than the adult haemoglobins, facilitating transfer of oxygen from the maternal to the fetal circulation.

Normally, the synthesis of α-like and β-like chains is balanced, although the mechanisms permitting this balance remain incompletely understood. An imbalance between the production of α and β chains is the pathophysiological basis of the thalassaemias. Disorders of haemoglobin structure may also arise in the absence of imbalance between the α and β globin chains, where mutated forms of globin are synthesized, and sickle cell anaemia is the principal example discussed in this chapter.

Thalassaemia

The thalassaemias are among the most common genetic disorders in the world and are also among the most intensively studied from a molecular perspective. Notwithstanding this, their treatment is frequently limited to supportive care, and they are responsible for significant disease worldwide, most especially in countries that are economically least able to meet this challenge (Figure 5.2).

The thalassaemias are divided into two main groups, the α-thalassaemias and the β-thalassaemias, depending on whether the defect lies in the synthesis of α- or β-globin chains, respectively. The pathophysiology reflects the impact of an imbalance in the expression of α- and β-globin chains. In β-thalassaemia, the excess α chains precipitate in the precursor red cells, leading to the premature destruction of these cells prior to their release from the bone marrow. This is *ineffective erythropoiesis*. In α-thalassaemia, excess β chains may also form tetramers, $\beta4$, an abnormal haemoglobin with a very high oxygen affinity termed HbH. In both forms of thalassaemia, precipitated excess globin chains also result in oxidative damage to the red cell membrane, with a consequent shortening of the red cell lifespan, giving a haemolytic element to their pathophysiology.

The resulting anaemia leads to an increased erythroid drive; this manifests in further ineffective erythropoiesis, and there is further expansion of the marrow into bones not typically used for haematopoiesis, and into the spleen. The long-term consequences of untreated thalassaemia may therefore

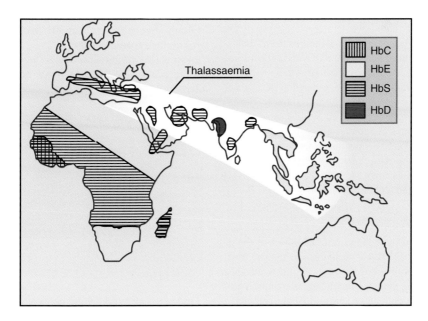

Figure 5.2 Areas of high prevalence for the major Hb variants (C, E, S, D) and thalassaemia, suggesting the most common ethnic backgrounds for individuals affected by these conditions.

include splenomegaly and bony deformities as well as chronic anaemia. The ineffective erythropoiesis also causes disruption to the hepcidin axis, with increased iron absorption from the gut. This, plus the requirement for transfusion in many of these patients, means that iron overload is a very significant aspect of the pathophysiology of the thalassaemias.

The severity of the disease will vary greatly according to the degree of globin chain imbalance. The clinical phenotypes of patients with thalassaemia are discussed in more detail below.

α-Thalassaemia

α-Thalassaemia is seen with the greatest frequency in people of South-East Asian and sub-Saharan African ethnicity. The prevalence in these countries is in the region of 20–30%. A relative resistance to *falciparum* malaria is thought to underlie the high prevalence in these areas. α-Thalassaemia is also prevalent in southern Europe and the Middle East, but sporadic cases have been reported in most racial groups.

Each chromosome 16 has an α-globin locus consisting of two α-globin genes, the embryonic ζ-globin gene plus the regulatory sequences essential for their normal expression. In most patients with α-thalassaemia, there is a deletion of one or more of the α-globin genes; there are occasional cases that are the consequence of non-deletional genetic defects.

α⁺ Thalassaemia trait

This is seen when an individual inherits the α⁺ thalassaemia allele from one parent and a normal chromosome 16 from the other parent. The most common genotype is termed $(\alpha\alpha/\alpha\text{-})^{3.7}$, a deletion of 3.7 kb of the affected chromosome. This and other α⁺ thalassaemia alleles are common in South-East Asia, the Mediterranean, sub-Saharan Africa, the Middle East and India. Affected individuals are asymptomatic, although they may have minor haematological changes such as slight reductions in mean cell volume (MCV) and mean cell haemoglobin (MCH).

α⁰ Thalassaemia trait

This is caused by deletion of both copies of the α-globin gene on a single chromosome 16. The most common deletion is termed $(\alpha\alpha/\text{-{-}})^{SEA}$, the South-East Asian deletion, though other deletions are found particularly in individuals of Thai and Filipino ethnicity; it is in these regions, plus the Mediterranean, that the α⁰ thalassaemia trait is typically found, with only rare

cases being seen in individuals of African ethnicity. Haematologically, the Hb is either normal or slightly reduced and the MCV and MCH are low. (Similar haematological changes are seen in homozygotes for the α⁺ thalassaemia allele, who also have a total of two α-globin genes deleted.)

Haemoglobin H disease

Inheritance of both the α⁺ and α⁰ thalassaemia alleles, leaving one functioning α-globin gene per cell, gives HbH disease, so termed because the excess β-globin chains form a tetramer termed HbH which can be detected by haemoglobin electrophoresis or haemoglobin high-performance liquid chromatography. HbH disease is therefore typically restricted to populations in which the α⁰ and α⁺ thalassaemia alleles are both found – South-East Asia and the Mediterranean. In northern Thailand, HbH disease is thought to affect approximately 1% of the population. HbH is unstable and precipitates as the erythrocytes age, forming rigid membrane-bound inclusions that are removed during the passage of affected red cells through the spleen. The damage to the membrane brought about by this removal results in a shortened red cell lifespan.

The clinical picture of HbH disease is very variable. Most patients are moderately affected, with a mild anaemia of 70–110 g/L, and markedly hypochromic microcytic red cell indices (Figure 5.3). Supravital staining of the blood film demonstrates cells with many HbH inclusions, giving a characteristic 'golf-ball' appearance (Figure 5.4). Affected patients will typically have splenomegaly.

Most patients will be transfusion independent, or require transfusions only at times of intercurrent infection. The clinical picture is therefore one of

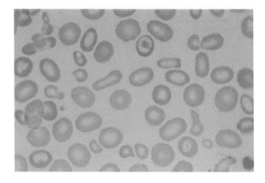

Figure 5.3 Blood film from a patient with HbH disease showing microcytosis, hypochromia, anisocytosis and poikilocytosis.

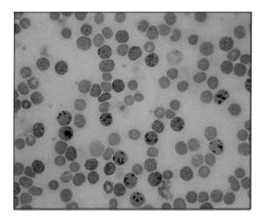

Figure 5.4 HbH inclusions seen on supravital staining with brilliant cresyl blue.

transfusion-independent thalassaemia, previously termed thalassaemia intermedia (see below).

Hb Bart's hydrops fetalis syndrome

This condition, in which no α-globin chains are synthesized at all, typically results in intrauterine death from hydrops. It occurs when there is homozygosity for an $α^0$ thalassaemia allele, and therefore occurs where $α^0$ thalassaemia trait is common. In the absence of the synthesis of α-globin chains in the developing fetus, the fetal β-like chain γ-globin forms tetramers known as Hb Bart's ($γ_4$). This haemoglobin is not suitable for oxygen transport and, although the embryonic haemoglobin Hb Portland ($ζ_2γ_2$) may persist in its expression for longer than is usual, infants with Hb Bart's are usually stillborn or die shortly after birth.

β-Thalassaemia

The World Health Organization estimates that 1.5% of the world's population are carriers of β-thalassaemia. The prevalence of the β-thalassaemia trait is particularly high in southern Europe (10–30%) and South-East Asia (5%), but it is also common in Africa, the Middle East, India, Pakistan and southern China. It has been suggested that the high prevalence of β-thalassaemia in these regions results from its protective effect against *Plasmodium falciparum* in heterozygotes.

While α-thalassaemia typically arises from gene deletions, β-thalassaemia usually results from a multiplicity of different single nucleotide substitutions, insertions or small deletions affecting the β-globin gene itself, its promoter or its upstream regulatory sequences. The prevalence of particular genetic

mutations varies among different ethnic groups. Analogous to the α-thalassaemias, $β^0$ thalassaemia describes a mutation that abolishes β-chain production from a given chromosome, while $β^+$ thalassaemia alleles allow some β-chain production, albeit at a reduced level. The $β^0$ type predominates in India and Pakistan and $β^+$ mutations predominate in Sardinia and Cyprus; both types are found in individuals whose ethnic background can be traced to Greece, the Middle East and Thailand. Because there is only a single copy of the β-globin gene on each copy of chromosome 11, the inheritance of β-thalassaemia is less complex than that of α-thalassaemia.

β-Thalassaemia trait

Most affected people with β-thalassaemia trait have a mutation affecting one copy of the β-globin gene (i.e. heterozygosity for a β-thalassaemia allele). They are typically asymptomatic. The Hb concentration is either normal or slightly reduced, and hypochromic and microcytic red cell indices are seen. Examination of the peripheral blood film may also show characteristic red cell abnormalities such as target cells and poikilocytes. In this regard, affected individuals have a clinical picture very similar to that of people with α-thalassaemia trait. However, a major clue to the diagnosis is the relatively increased expression of δ-globin expression. This occurs from alleles in which β-globin expression is reduced or absent. The increased δ-chains will join the normally produced α-globin chains to form HbA$_2$ ($α_2δ_2$). Typically in β-thalassaemia trait, HbA$_2$ levels will be raised above the normal range to 3.5–7.0%, and this provides a useful laboratory diagnostic clue to the presence of beta thalassaemia trait (Figure 5.5). Some patients also show slightly increased HbF levels, in the range of 1–5%.

Homozygous β-thalassaemia

The exact nature of the mutations affecting the β-globin cluster plus the impact of various genetic modifiers will determine the phenotype of patients with defects of β-globin on both copies of chromosome 11. In the more severe cases, marked anaemia develops between the second and 12th months of life following the physiological switch from expression of the fetal γ-globin chain to reliance on the adult β-globin chain. At this point, patients become transfusion dependent. In other cases, a more moderate anaemia is seen, presenting after the age of 1–2 years and requiring transfusion only intermittently or in the context of intercurrent infection.

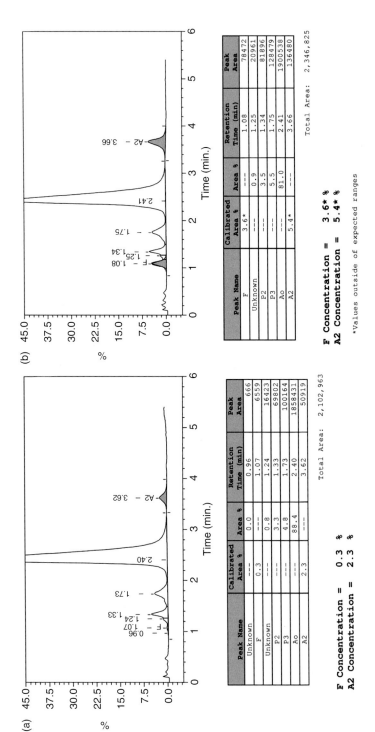

(a)

Peak Name	Calibrated Area %	Area %	Retention Time (min)	Peak Area
Unknown	---	0.0	0.96	666
F	0.3	---	1.07	6559
Unknown	---	0.8	1.24	16423
P2	---	3.3	1.33	69802
P3	---	4.8	1.73	100164
Ao	---	88.4	2.40	1858431
A2	2.3	---	3.62	50919

Total Area: 2,102,963

F Concentration =   0.3 %
A2 Concentration =   2.3 %

(b)

Peak Name	Calibrated Area %	Area %	Retention Time (min)	Peak Area
F	3.6*	---	1.08	78472
Unknown	---	0.9	1.25	20961
P2	---	3.5	1.34	81896
P3	---	5.5	1.75	128479
Ao	---	81.0	2.41	1900538
A2	5.4*	---	3.66	136480

Total Area: 2,346,825

F Concentration =   3.6* %
A2 Concentration =   5.4* %

*Values outside of expected ranges

Figure 5.5 High-performance liquid chromatography (HPLC) is the usual laboratory method used for the initial investigation of patients with haemoglobin disorders. After lysing the red cells, the haemoglobins in solution are passed across a chromatography column, and can be separated out. Panel A shows a normal HPLC trace; panel B shows a typical trace from an individual with β-thalassaemia trait – note the increased HbA_2 peak.

Clinical classification of the thalassaemias

The molecular basis for the thalassaemias is very diverse, and even in cases where the precise molecular defect is known, the impact of genetic modifiers may make it difficult to predict the exact clinical phenotype. Therefore, a clinical classification of the thalassaemias allows a description of the patient's phenotype irrespective of the exact molecular details of their underlying condition. Historically the terms *minor*, *intermedia* and *major* were used to classify thalassaemia, with minor equating to thalassaemia trait, thalassaemia intermedia suggesting a more significant globin imbalance requiring transfusion in the context of intercurrent illness, and thalassaemia major describing patients with an absolute reliance on regular transfusion. However, a simpler classification of non-transfusion-dependent and transfusion-dependent thalassaemia is now typically used.

Transfusion dependent thalassaemia and β-thalassaemia major are essentially synonymous, with β-globin synthesis so severely reduced that transfusion is essential for survival. The ongoing production of fetal haemoglobin into infancy permits these patients to survive *ex utero*, unlike those with complete loss of α-globin expression. However, with the progressive loss of fetal haemoglobin in the first few months of life, the infant becomes profoundly anaemic and would be unlikely to survive without transfusional support.

For patients in this situation, a transfusion programme is essential to avoid the consequences of severe anaemia. The severely ineffective erythropoiesis leads to increased signalling through the HIF/epo pathway. However, since this cannot generate normal mature red cells to provide negative feedback and to turn off epo signalling, the consequence is ongoing increased epo signalling, leading to ongoing erythroid expansion in the bone marrow. Eventually, the unchecked marrow expansion leads to expansion and deformation of the bones, as well as extramedullary erythropoiesis and splenomegaly.

Clinical course and complications of transfusion-dependent thalassaemia

As well as the anaemia, splenomegaly and bony deformities already discussed, transfusion-dependent thalassaemia is also characterized by the general features of hypermetabolic states, such as growth retardation. Iron absorption from the gut is increased (see Chapter 3) and, in conjunction with iron loading from red cell transfusions, this contributes to marked iron overload. Iron deposition occurs in the myocardium, which can cause congestive cardiac failure and potentially fatal arrhythmias; in the liver, leading to cirrhosis; in the pancreas, causing diabetes mellitus; and in other endocrine organs, leading to delayed puberty and delay or failure of the development of secondary sexual characteristics. While untransfused patients are likely to succumb to their anaemia in the first decade of life, transfused patients have their life expectancy reduced by the development of iron overload, and controlling iron loading is therefore a key goal in the treatment of patients with transfusion-dependent thalassaemia.

Treatment of transfusion-dependent thalassaemia

Transfusions (with extended red cell phenotyping; see also Chapter 15) are planned to maintain the pretransfusion Hb concentration at 90–100 g/L or above, with a post-transfusion Hb concentration of 130–140 g/L. With this treatment, children with transfusion-dependent thalassaemia are able to grow and mature normally. If the spleen is considerably enlarged, with evidence that it is also trapping transfused red cells and increasing transfusion requirements, splenectomy can be performed. Splenectomy may also be considered if there is thrombocytopenia or leucopenia secondary to pooling of the blood volume in the enlarged spleen.

An important aspect of treatment is the reduction of tissue damage caused by secondary iron overload. Historically, this required the use of desferrioxamine, an iron chelator that could be administered only parenterally and required subcutaneous infusion treatment over several hours on 5 days of the week. Unsurprisingly for such a burdensome treatment, compliance can be problematic. Oral iron chelators such as deferasirox and deferiprone are now used, with excellent outcomes. Effective iron chelation is critical to the long-term health of patients with transfusion-dependent thalassaemia, and may also be needed in patients with non-transfusion-dependent thalassaemia, because of the intermittent transfusion requirements and the effects of increased iron absorption from the gut (Figure 5.6).

More radical and curative approaches have also been taken for patients with transfusion-dependent

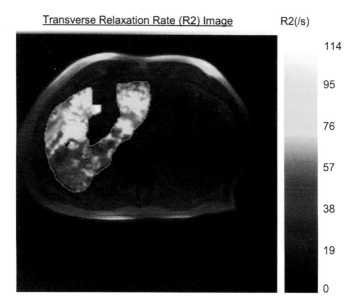

Figure 5.6 The Ferriscan™ is a form of magnetic resonance imaging, specifically developed for giving a non-invasive estimate of liver iron concentration. The scan shown is from a patient with transfusion-dependent thalassaemia major who takes regular chelation. There is a mild increase in hepatic iron at 2.9 mg/g dry tissue (reference range 0.17–1.8).

thalassaemia. Haematopoietic stem cell transplantation has been performed in many patients, although the limiting factor is frequently the availability of human leucocyte antigen (HLA)-matched donors. Although the morbidity and mortality of the procedure in young patients (treated before the development of end-organ damage caused by iron deposition) are low, they are not negligible; the risks of the procedure therefore have to be weighed against the prospect of decades of treatment by blood transfusion and iron chelation, and a personalized treatment plan must be created for each patient. In older patients, transplantation has proved less attractive an option, largely because of the higher procedure-related morbidity and mortality.

More experimental treatments include gene therapy. Patients' own haematopoietic stem cells are harvested, then genetically modified, either with lentiviral vector introduction of the normal β-globin gene or with CRISPR-cas9 gene editing. These edited haematopoietic stem cells are then reinfused to the patient, and home to the bone marrow to reconstitute normal haematopoiesis. While problems remain with these still novel techniques, gene therapy remains a long-term goal for patients with transfusion-dependent thalassaemia.

Genetic counselling and antenatal diagnosis of transfusion-dependent β-thalassaemia

When a pregnant woman is found to have an abnormality in the synthesis or structure of Hb, her partner must also be investigated. If there is a risk of serious clinical disease in the fetus, antenatal diagnosis should be offered. Antenatal diagnosis can be made early during pregnancy from an analysis of chorionic villus DNA (at 9–12 weeks) or amniocyte DNA (at 13–16 weeks), or later using DNA from blood obtained from an 18–20-week-old fetus. Newer techniques focus on the non-invasive analysis of fetal DNA in the maternal circulation.

Structural haemoglobin variants

Over 1000 abnormal haemoglobin variants have been reported, but most are rare and only a few lead to clinical or haematological manifestations. Those which do lead to clinical problems, however, can have

Table 5.1 Different clinical and haematological abnormalities associated with some structural haemoglobin variants.

Variant	Clinical and haematological abnormalities
HbS	Recurrent painful crises and chronic haemolytic anaemia, both related to sickling of red cells on deoxygenation
HbC	Chronic haemolytic anaemia due to reduced red cell deformability on deoxygenation; deoxygenated HbC is less soluble than deoxygenated HbA
Hb Köln, Hb Hammersmith	Spontaneous or drug-induced haemolytic anaemia caused by instability of the Hb and consequent intracellular precipitation
HbM Boston, HbM Saskatoon	Cyanosis reflecting congenital methaemoglobinaemia as a consequence of a substitution near or in the haem pocket
Hb Chesapeake, Hb Radcliffe	Hereditary polycythaemia caused by increased O_2 affinity of the haemoglobin variant
Hb Kansas	Anaemia and cyanosis caused by decreased O_2 affinity of the haemoglobin variant
Hb Constant Spring, Hb Lepore, HbE	Thalassaemia-like syndrome caused by decreased rate of synthesis of abnormal globin chain
Hb Indianapolis	Thalassaemia-like syndrome caused by marked instability of Hb

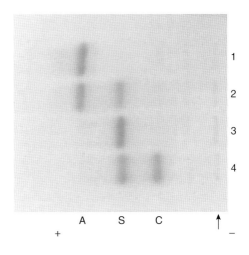

Figure 5.7 Electrophoresis of haemolysates on cellulose acetate (pH 8.5). The arrow marks the site of application of the haemolysate. (1) Normal adult. (2) Individual with sickle cell trait; 35% of the Hb consists of HbS and most of the remainder is HbA. (3) Patient with sickle cell anaemia; most of the Hb is S and there is no HbA. (4) Compound heterozygote for HbS and HbC. This results in a sickling disorder that is often milder than that in homozygotes for HbS.

abnormal haemoglobin variants are detected by high-performance liquid chromatography (HPLC), using a similar principle (Figure 5.8).

The most common structural Hb variant is haemoglobin S (HbS). This globin variant, and the important clinical entity of sickle cell anaemia, are discussed in the following section.

Haemoglobin S

Sickle cell anaemia has been described as the first 'molecular disease'. It was the first condition in which a defect in a specific protein was determined to be causative (by Linus Pauling and colleagues in 1948), with the specific amino acid change being defined in 1956. A mutation in the β-globin gene results in the charged glutamic acid residue in position 6 of the normal β-chain being replaced by an uncharged valine molecule. The interaction of sickle β-globin chains with normal α-globin chains forms the abnormal haemoglobin, HbS. When deoxygenated, HbS is much less soluble than deoxygenated HbA, and HbS molecules polymerize, eventually forming long fibres

serious and wide-ranging implications for health and life expectancy.

The majority of structural Hb variants are the consequence of a point mutation with a single amino acid substitution in the affected globin chain (e.g. HbS, HbE, HbC and HbD). The spectrum of clinical and haematological abnormalities that can be caused by such abnormal haemoglobins is summarized in Table 5.1. When the amino acid substitution results in an overall change in the charge of the haemoglobin molecule, its migration in a voltage gradient is altered and this can be demonstrated by standard electrophoretic techniques, with the speed of migration being characteristic for each abnormal haemoglobin (Figure 5.7). More commonly in clinical practice,

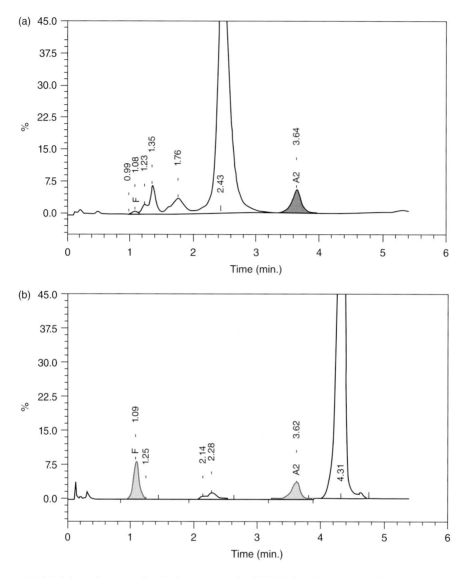

Figure 5.8 (a) High-performance liquid chromatography (HPLC) showing a trace with no variant haemoglobins but an increased peak at the retention time of HbA₂, consistent with β-thalassaemia trait. (b) HPLC trace showing a variant haemoglobin with the retention time of HbS.

(tactoids; Figure 5.9). These result in the deformation of the cell into the well-recognized sickle shape (Figure 5.10). Red cells from heterozygotes for HbS sickle only at much lower pO₂ values than those from homozygotes, and do not usually sickle *in vivo*.

The sickle mutation occurs particularly in patients of African ethnicity as well as those from parts of the Middle East and southern Indian (see Figure 5.2).

Its prevalence in these areas varies from very low values to 40% of the population. In black Americans, the prevalence is 8%. The distribution of the βˢ gene corresponds to areas in which *falciparum* malaria has been endemic; its persistence at high frequency in these areas reflects the relative resistance of heterozygotes to severe *falciparum* malaria during early childhood.

asymptomatic as the red cells do not sickle until the O_2 saturation falls below 40%, a level that is rarely reached in venous blood. However, spontaneous haematuria may occur occasionally because of microvascular infarctions in the renal medulla. Renal papillary necrosis may rarely occur and there is often an impaired ability to concentrate urine in older individuals. There is also an expanding literature on the possibility of an increased risk of exertional sudden death in athletes with sickle cell trait compared with controls, though the nature and mechanism remain the subject of investigation.

Sickle cell anaemia

People who are homozygous for sickle β-globin are described as having sickle cell anaemia. Their red cells contain almost exclusively HbS and no HbA; there is a small but variable percentage of fetal haemoglobin ($\alpha_2\gamma_2$) n, as well as some HbA_2 ($\alpha_2\delta_2$).

The cells may sickle at the O_2 tension normally found in venous blood. Sickled red cells then occlude the microvasculature, with poor downstream perfusion and oxygenation. They may be lysed directly in the circulation, where the resulting free haemoglobin scavenges nitric oxide; this in turn promotes vascular endothelial dysfunction and further vaso-occlusion. Sickled cells have also been shown to have abnormal interaction with endothelial cells, promoting an inflammatory reaction and inappropriate activation of the coagulation cascade. Thus, although sickling of red cells due to the poor solubility of deoxygenated HbS is the ultimate basis of sickle cell anaemia, the disease is now recognized to be much more complex than the simple obstruction of the microvasculature by sickled cells. Our understanding of the pathophysiology of this condition is still far from complete.

Initially, there are cycles of sickling and reversal of sickling as the red cells are repeatedly deoxygenated and reoxygenated within the circulation. Eventually, as membrane damage accumulates, irreversibly sickled cells are formed. Both unsickled and sickled red cells containing deoxygenated HbS are less deformable than normal red cells and this results in a chronic, principally extravascular haemolytic anaemia. The Hb usually varies between 60 and 90 g/L, but the symptoms referable to the anaemia itself are milder than expected from the Hb levels, as HbS has a reduced affinity for O_2 (i.e. the O_2 dissociation curve is shifted to the right).

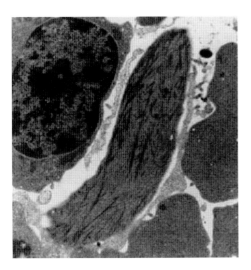

Figure 5.9 Electron micrograph of a sickled red cell from a homozygote for HbS showing fibres of polymerized deoxygenated HbS running along the long axis of the cell.

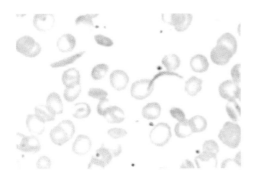

Figure 5.10 Two sickle-shaped red cells and some partially sickled red cells from the blood film of a patient with sickle cell anaemia (homozygote for HbS).

Sickle cell trait

Patients who are carriers of the sickle cell mutation (having one normal β-globin gene and one bearing the β^s mutation) are described as having sickle cell trait. Their red cells contain between 20% and 45% HbS, the rest being mainly HbA. (The HbS is less than 50% mainly because mutant β-chains [β^s] have a lower affinity than normal β-chains to associate with α-chains.) Individuals with sickle cell trait are usually

Diagnosis

Sickled cells are invariably present on the blood films of patients with HbSS (see Figure 5.10). The diagnosis of HbSS is made by finding: (i) a positive result with a screening test for HbS; and (ii) a peak at an appropriate position on an HPLC trace, confirmed by isoelectric focusing or haemoglobin electrophoresis. The screening tests for HbS-containing red cells are based on the decreased solubility of deoxygenated HbS; they involve the development of turbidity after addition to a lysis buffer containing a reducing agent such as sodium dithionite (sickle solubility test). Heterozygotes for HbS also give a positive result with these screening tests, but would be expected to show both HbA and HbS on HPLC and/or haemoglobin electrophoresis.

The clinical picture of sickle cell anaemia is highly variable (Table 5.2), reflecting the impact of genetic modifiers. Patients with hereditary persistence of fetal haemoglobin, for example, have a much milder phenotype than those patients in whom HbF is appropriately silenced. The coinheritance of

α-thalassaemia trait, which will reduce the MCH, can also ameliorate the symptoms of sickle cell anaemia.

Typically, individuals with sickle cell anaemia have crises superimposed on their chronic haemolytic state, sometimes precipitated by infection, cold or dehydration but sometimes with no obvious precipitant at all. Crises frequently take the form of acute vaso-occlusive painful episodes, which can affect any part of the body. In young children, a classic acute painful presentation is with dactylitis, or the 'hand–foot syndrome', in which there is occlusion of the arteries to the metacarpals and metatarsals (Figure 5.11) and consequent painful swelling of the hands and feet.

Aside from painful crises, sickle cell anaemia also has wide-ranging complications that can affect any organ of the body. In the central nervous system, cerebral infarction occurs in approximately 10% of patients under the age of 20, and is a cause of significant morbidity in sickle cell patients. It has been found that children with an increased velocity of blood flow in the major cerebral vessels are at particular risk of stroke, and transcranial Doppler studies now constitute an important part of the screening of paediatric patients with sickle cell anaemia. Children with high-risk transcranial Doppler readings receive prophylactic treatment in the form of regular transfusions to minimize their risk of stroke. Haemorrhagic stroke may also be seen, but is more common in older patients.

Cardiorespiratory presentations include the acute chest syndrome (typically with dyspnoea, falling oxygen saturations and chest radiograph abnormalities),

Table 5.2 Clinical manifestations of sickle cell anaemia.

Acute complications	Chronic complications
Painful vaso-occlusive crises	Chronic haemolytic anaemia and consequent cholelithiasis
Acute chest syndrome	Avascular necrosis (especially of the femoral head)
Cerebral infarction, intracranial haemorrhage	Chronic leg ulcers
Splenic sequestration syndrome; rarely, hepatic sequestration	Osteomyelitis (*Salmonella, Staphylococcus*)
Priapism	Chronic pulmonary disease and pulmonary hypertension
Aplastic crises caused by parvovirus infection	Haematuria, proteinuria, chronic kidney disease
	Proliferative sickle retinopathy (more common in HbSC disease)
	Pregnancy: increased peripartum fetal loss, preterm births, babies small for gestational age

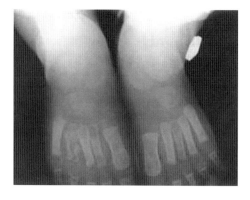

Figure 5.11 An X-ray of the feet of a child with sickle cell anaemia 2 weeks after the onset of hand–foot syndrome, showing necrosis of the right fourth metatarsal.

Box 5.1 **Haematological emergency: the acute chest syndrome in sickle cell disease**

The acute chest syndrome is one of the most feared complications of sickle cell disease,. It arises from the development of sickling within the pulmonary vasculature, which limits the degree of gas exchange possible at the affected sites. This results in worsening hypoxia – itself a prompt for further sickling. The acute chest syndrome is therefore characterized by a downward spiral of hypoxia, sickling, shunting within the pulmonary vessels and worsening hypoxia; if untreated, it can lead to death.

It may be initiated by infection or may arise in the context of a painful crisis affecting the chest, back or ribs – often associated with a degree of hypoventilation. Clinically, a chest crisis is suspected in any patient with a sickling disorder with (i) falling oxygen saturations, (ii) respiratory symptoms (e.g. cough, dyspnoea), and (iii) new infiltrates on a chest x-ray (though these may take time to develop). Clearly, this clinical picture overlaps significantly with that of lower respiratory tract infection, and empiric antibiotic therapy is usually given. If the patient's oxygen saturations continue to fall despite antibiotic treatment and supplemental oxygen therapy, intervention for presumed chest crisis is needed.

Addressing the underlying pathology is central to management of the acute chest syndrome, and a key aim is to reduce the percentage of HbS within the patient's blood. Normally in patients with sickle cell disease, this is near to 100%. Bringing the HbS% down to <30% arrests the sickling process and improves oxygenation of the tissues. This reduction in the HbS% usually requires an exchange transfusion – the removal of the patient's own red cells, and replacement with non-HbS-containing donor blood. A significant reduction in HbS usually requires an exchange of several units of blood, with the exact requirement being established using the patient's calculated blood volume, resting Hb and pre-exchange HbS%. In most centres, the exchange is peformed using an apheresis machine (see Chapter 12) but manual exchange can be performed if needed in an emergency. A simple top-up transfusion is unlikely to reduce the HbS% significantly, but may on occasions be useful in early chest crisis, or as a holding measure while automated exchange is set up. While the clinical course is highly variable, some patients deteriorate rapidly and may require intubation and ventilatory support.

---

which can be fatal if untreated. This syndrome and its emergency management are discussed in Box 5.1.

More chronic cardiorespiratory complications include the development of pulmonary hypertension and right heart failure, with a number of contributory factors including thromboembolism, multiple episodes of acute chest syndrome and endothelial dysfunction from nitric oxide scavenging by free haemoglobin.

As with all chronic haemolytic anaemias, there is an increase in the incidence of pigment gallstones. Additional hepatic complications include vaso-occlusion of the hepatic sinusoids, which can result in marked cholestasis. Renal complications include renal papillary necrosis as a result of infarction. Renal failure is thought to develop in up to one-quarter of patients with HbSS and is caused by a combination of cortical and medullary infarction, glomerular sclerosis, tubular damage and infection. Detection of proteinuria in patients with sickle cell disease can be useful in attempting to delay the onset of serious renal disease. Priapism is another common problem.

Young children can develop potentially life-threatening acute splenic sequestration – a crisis caused by the rapid and extensive trapping of red cells in the spleen, leading to profound anaemia, massive splenomegaly, reduced blood volume and hypovolaemic shock. Repeated splenic infarcts lead to functional hyposplenism, with an increased risk of infection, particularly from encapsulated organisms. Infection used to be the most common cause of mortality in paediatric sickle cell patients, though the use of prophylactic antibiotics and asplenic vaccination protocols has had a major impact on this.

In terms of musculoskeletal and skin complications, patients may develop larger infarcts affecting the bones, with avascular necrosis of the femoral head being a potential complication. Osteomyelitis is another recognized complication and is classically found to be caused by *Salmonella typhi*. Chronic leg ulcers are often seen (Figure 5.12) and can be very difficult to treat.

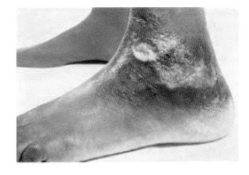

Figure 5.12 A chronic leg ulcer with increased pigmentation of the surrounding skin in a woman with sickle cell anaemia.

A proliferative sickle retinopathy may develop and can lead to blindness from vitreous haemorrhage and retinal detachment; retinopathy is more common in compound heterozygotes for HbS and HbC (i.e. in HbSC disease) than in sickle cell anaemia, and results from hypoxaemic conditions downstream of occluded vessels.

Aplastic crises caused by parvovirus infection may occur (see Chapter 11), as may an exacerbation of the anaemia resulting from secondary folic acid deficiency (see Chapter 3).

Treatment

The management of sickle cell anaemia includes the following.

- Management of the increased infection risk by immunization with pneumococcal, *Haemophilus influenzae* type b (Hib) and meningococcal vaccines, plus treatment with prophylactic penicillin. This is particularly critical for children, but continues lifelong. Non-immune patients should also receive hepatitis B vaccine in case many transfusions are required.
- Administration of folic acid daily to prevent secondary folate deficiency.
- Avoidance of factors precipitating painful crises such as dehydration, hypoxia and circulatory stasis.
- Active treatment for bacterial infections that may precipitate or have precipitated crises.
- Treatment of painful crises with oral or intravenous fluids and analgesics, including opiates when necessary.
- Early detection of the acute chest syndrome (blood gas measurements and chest x-ray), with the administration of oxygen and respiratory support where appropriate. Exchange transfusions are often needed to lower the patient's HbS levels and limit ongoing sickling.
- Blood transfusion when necessary. Careful top-up transfusion may be indicated for sequestration and aplastic crises, and exchange transfusions are useful in certain situations, particularly in severe acute chest syndrome (see Box 5.1) and in cases where there is evidence of neurological damage. A chronic transfusion programme may also be initiated in children at high risk of stroke (i.e. when transcranial Doppler studies show increased middle artery blood flow velocity) to suppress the patient's own endogenous erythroid drive, and

thereby to reduce the HbS content of blood. This has been shown in clinical trials to have a major impact on reducing the incidence of stroke, and newer studies also suggest that treatment with hydroxycarbamide may have a similar protective effect in selected patients. As in the case of transfusion-dependent thalassaemia, patients who are regularly transfused for prolonged periods (>1–2 years) must receive iron chelators to prevent iron overload. Transfusion may also be required during pregnancy in patients with frequent crises or a poor obstetric history. Rarely, patients with sickle cell disease may suffer the complication of hyperhaemolysis following transfusion – a haemolytic transfusion reaction (see Chapter 15) in which the patient's own red cells are lysed as well as the transfused donor cells. Although the pathogenesis of this potentially life-threatening complication is not well understood, the anti-CD20 monoclonal antibody rituximab and the complement inhibitor eculizumab have been found to be clinically useful in managing it.

In symptomatic patients with sickling disorders, there is evidence to support the use of the strategies to increase the proportion of haemoglobin contributed by HbF. Since the fetal γ-globin chains cannot be incorporated into the polymerized sickle haemoglobin, the presence of HbF is therefore able to inhibit the sickling process. Sickle cell patients with coinherited inappropriate expression of γ-globin after infancy (known as hereditary persistence of fetal haemoglobin, HPFH) have a much milder phenotype than those in whom fetal globin is silenced normally. Much research effort has therefore gone into understanding the mechanisms by which fetal globin is silenced (Box 5.2), with a view to its therapeutic reactivation. The current pharmacological intervention to try to elevate HbF expression is long-term therapy with the ribonucleotide reductase inhibitor hydroxycarbamide; this increases the synthesis of HbF to a limited extent by means that are incompletely understood, and indeed modes of action other than HbF induction have been proposed to explain its therapeutic benefits. Whatever the true basis of its effect, it can yield a significant reduction in the frequency of crises, and also significantly reduces mortality in patients with sickle cell disease. It is therefore widely used in patients who suffer at least one painful crisis per year, as well as those who have suffered chest crises or other complications which adversely affect their quality of life.

Box 5.2 Reactivating silenced fetal haemoglobin

The β-globinopathies present a major burden of morbidity and mortality worldwide. All present clinically as the normal haemoglobin 'switch' from HbF to HbA takes place in the first few months after birth; patients with hereditary persistence of fetal haemoglobin are therefore largely protected from the most severe clinical manifestations.

The possibility of reactivating the normal γ-globin gene alongside the defective β-globin gene has long been considered an attractive therapeutic option. Yet, as with all genes, the details of how its expression is activated and silenced in a developmental stage-specific manner remain poorly understood.

A significant step forward was made in 2008 with the discovery of the role of BCL11a, a DNA-binding protein. Sequence variants in the gene for BCL11a were found to be frequently implicated in patients with hereditary persistence of fetal hemoglobin, and subsequent work demonstrated that high levels of BCL11a were found only in mature red cells. Moreover, the experimental downregulation of BCL11a is able to reinstate high levels of HbF production, with clinically relevant amelioration of the haematological phenotype in animal models of sickle cell anaemia. Small-scale clinical trials have reported successful treatment of patients with sickle cell disease and transfusion-dependent thalassaemia by inactivating a transcriptional enhancer which is normally responsible for BCL11a transcription in red cells. By this means, clinically useful reactivation of HbF has been achieved. Such treatments are complex and expensive and are currently unavailable to many patients with major haemoglobin disorders. Agents such as hydroxycarbamide, which can achieve modest elevations of HbF synthesis with good clinical effect, are widely available, however, and are increasingly used in the treatment of sickle cell anaemia.

The clinical response to hydroxycarbamide varies from patient to patient, and second-line therapies may also be required. Newer agents approved for use in these settings include the monoclonal antibody crizanlizumab, which blocks P-selectin. By reducing the adhesion between platelets and neutrophils and activated endothelial cells, this agent has been shown to reduce the frequency of painful vaso-occlusive crises in sickle cell disease.

Other agents under active investigation include voxelotor and L-glutamine. Voxelotor effects an allosteric change in the structure of HbS to increase its oxygen affinity. Since it is deoxygenated HbS which polymerizes and causes the sickling of red cells, voxelotor impacts directly on the pathophysiology of the disease, and has been shown to reduce the degree of haemolysis seen in patients with HbSS. L-glutamine is thought to work by reducing the degree of oxidative stress experienced by the red cell, and may reduce the frequency of painful crises in patients with sickle cell disease.

Curative strategies do exist for sickle cell disease. As with transfusion-dependent thalassaemia, bone marrow transplantation is currently the only curative treatment, though the decision to proceed with transplantation is not always straightforward. Patients with a suitably severe phenotype must be identified prior to the onset of organ damage; consequently, most transplants have been undertaken in children, with the best results seen in those with matched sibling donors, though transplant is increasingly undertaken in adults too. Typical overall survival rates are 90–97%, with event-free survival being near 85%. The potential risks of the procedure need to be weighed carefully against the implications of chronic disease for each young patient when deciding on an appropriate treatment strategy.

Technical advances in the genetic modification of haematopoietic stem cells also raise the possibility of autologous stem cell transplantion in sickle cell disease using cells subject to 'gene editing' *ex vivo*. Successful CRISPR modification of autologous haematopoietic stem cells used for transplantation into patients with sickle cell disease has been reported, with the target for modification being a red cell-specific enhancer for BCL11a (see Box 5.2).

Haemoglobins E and C

There are many haemoglobin variants other than HbS with clinical consequences. Among the most common are HbE and HbC, both of which result from single amino acid substitutions in the β-chains.

HbE is a structural variant of β-globin in which a missense mutation creates a new splice site at the end of the first intron–exon boundary. Patients with HbE therefore have a reduction in normally spliced β-globin mRNA, with subsequent reduction in the amount of β-globin produced from the affected allele, rather like a form of β-thalassaemia. Heterozygotes have about 20–30% HbE, are asymptomatic and are usually not anaemic, although they do have a low

MCV consistent with the thalassaemia-like patho-physiology. Homozygous patients are characterized by mild anaemia, a low MCV and many circulating target cells. The main clinical significance of this globin variant, however, is its coinheritance with β-thalassaemia. As HbE is very common in South-East Asia (being found in about 50% of the population in some parts of Thailand), compound heterozygosity for Eβ-thalassaemia is not unusual. Such patients have highly variable clinical presentations, but the more severely affected have a transfusion-dependent thalassaemia phenotype.

HbC is the consequence of a glutamine-to-lysine substitution in the β-globin chain, producing a positively charged haemoglobin molecule. When coinherited with a sickle allele, the resulting HbSC gives a sickling phenotype, although with some specific features (such as a more marked propensity to proliferative retinopathy). HbC is also seen in homozygosity; here the haemoglobin does not polymerize as it does in HbSS, but it can crystallize, with a resulting reduction in the flexibility of the red cell and in its survival. Abnormalities of potassium handling within HbCC red cells also contribute to the phenotype. Homozygous patients have a mild anaemia, low MCV, splenomegaly and many target cells in their blood film (Figure 5.13), while heterozygotes tend to be clinically asymptomatic.

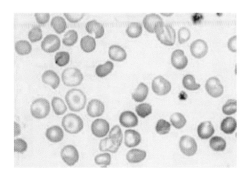

Figure 5.13 Target cells and irregularly contracted cells in the blood film of a homozygote for HbC.

HbC is found in patients of West African origin, where the incidence may be as high as 7% of the population in Nigeria and 22% in northern Ghana.

While HbS, HbE and HbC are among the most common structural defects in the globins, many others exist, each with its own impact on the normal structure and function of haemoglobin. An understanding of the molecular nature of these disorders has been crucial to appreciating their pathophysiology and is likely to be of benefit in developing effective therapies in the future.

6

An introduction to haematological malignancies

LEARNING OBJECTIVES

After reading this chapter, you should be able to:

✓ describe the broad framework by which haematological malignances are classified

✓ understand that the cell of origin is important in classification

✓ recognize the importance of genetic abnormalities in the aetiology and classification of haematological malignances

✓ understand how staging systems are used in haematological malignancies

✓ describe the general approach to treatment and supportive care.

Haematological malignances are clonal disorders that derive from a single cell located in either the bone marrow or the peripheral lymphoid tissue. In the UK, approximately 7% of malignant disorders are haematological cancers although they are disproportionately represented in the young (the most common childhood cancer, for example, is acute lymphoblastic leukaemia).

Cancers result from the accumulation of genetic mutations within a cell. Haematological malignancies tend to have fewer mutations in comparison to some solid tumours (for example, acute myeloid leukaemia (AML) typically has approximately four mutations in comparison to lung cancer which has an average of approximately 125). Malignant change in cells arises as a multistep process, with the serial acquisition of mutations, each of which confers a selective growth advantage. This may occur by linear evolution (whereby the final clone harbours all the mutations that arose during evolution) or by branching evolution, where there are multiple different subclones, each of which shares a common ancestral cell. Treatments may lead to selective killing of some subclones but allow others to survive, partially explaining why some patients may relapse.

The genes involved in the development of cancer are classically divided into two groups: oncogenes and tumour suppressor genes.

Oncogenes are genes which promote the development of malignancies as a consequence of gain-of-function mutations or an inappropriate expression pattern. Mutations in these genes typically affect the processes of cell signalling, cell differentiation and cell survival. A common subset of genes which are mutated produce tyrosine kinase enzymes, which phosphorylate proteins on tyrosine residues and are

Haematology Lecture Notes, Eleventh Edition. Deborah Hay, Andrew King and Michael Desborough.
© 2023 John Wiley & Sons Ltd. Published 2023 by John Wiley & Sons Ltd.
Companion website: www.wiley.com/go/Hay/Haematology/11e

important mediators of intracellular signalling. Examples include ABL1 (in chronic myeloid leukaemia), JAK2 (in myeloproliferative neoplasms), FLT3 (in AML) and Bruton tyrosine kinase in chronic lymphocytic leukaemia (CLL). These will be discussed in further detail in the disease-specific chapters which follow.

The other main class of genes involved in the development of haematological disease are *tumour suppressor genes*. These normally control a cell during division and replication through the cell cycle. If they acquire loss-of-function mutations, usually by point mutation or deletion, this may lead to malignant transformation. *p53* is the best known tumour suppressor gene, and plays an important role in many haematological cancers.

Chromosomal abnormalities

A normal somatic cell has 46 chromosomes. These occur in pairs and are numbered 1–22 in decreasing size order; there are in addition two sex chromosomes, XX in females and XY in males. A *karyotype* is the term used to describe the chromosomes derived from a cell undergoing mitosis, with specific conventions determining how the complement of chromosomes is described (Table 6.1).

Characteristic chromosomal abnormalities such as those given in Table 6.1 are a feature of both myeloid and lymphoid haematological malignancies. Often, the more complex the karyotypic abnormalities, the more difficult it is to treat the underlying disease.

Translocations, especially common in haematological malignancy compared with solid tumours, may contribute to malignant change in two ways.

- Fusion of parts of two distinct genes to generate a new chimeric fusion gene which encodes a dysfunctional or novel fusion protein (for example, BCR-ABL1 in chronic myeloid leukaemia and B-lymphoblastic leukaemia; Figure 6.1).
- Overexpression of a normal cellular gene – for example, overexpression of *MYC* in Burkitt lymphoma (Figure 6.2) through changes to its normal transcriptional regulation.

Chromosomal deletions, for example –7 or del(7q) in AML, are thought to lead to malignant change through loss of a tumour suppressor gene or other cell

Table 6.1 Karyotype naming conventions.

Karyotype shorthand	Meaning
p	Denotes the short arm of the chromosome
q	Denotes the long arm of the chromosome
+	Gain of a chromosome, e.g. +8, trisomy 8
–	Loss of a chromosome, e.g. – 7, monosomy 7
del	Loss of part of a chromosome, e.g. del(7q)
t	Translocation, e.g. t(9;22), a translocation between chromosomes 9 and 22. The larger chromosome is shown first in brackets
inv	A chromosomal inversion, e.g. inv(16), where part of the chromosome is orientated in the wrong direction

cycle regulator, although the exact mechanisms often remain unclear. Chromosomal duplications (for example, trisomy 12 in chronic lymphocytic leukaemia or trisomy 8 in AML) occur commonly although their underlying mechanism is poorly understood.

Epigenetic alterations

Mutations causing cancer may also occur in genes which are responsible for the regulation transcription, for example through altering DNA methylation (*DNMT3A* and *TET2*), or the acetylation or methylation of histone proteins around which DNA is packaged as chromatin (e.g. *ASXL1* and *EZH2*). Genes encoding enzymes that mediate the splicing of genes (for example, *SF3B1*, *SRSF2*, *U2AF1*) are also recurrently mutated in myeloid malignancies. The mechanisms by which these changes lead to the development of cancer are complex, since the changes to epigenetic regulation which result from their mutation will affect the expression of a large number of genes.

Identification of the genetic and molecular abnormalities in both myeloid and lymphoid diseases sheds light on their underlying pathogenesis but also provides valuable diagnostic information and potential therapeutic options via targeted therapy.

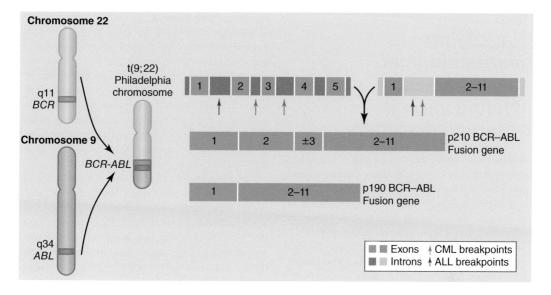

Figure 6.1 Illustration of the translocation between chromosomes 22 and 9 leading to the formation of a novel oncogene *BCR-ABL*. Note that a variation of the same translocation occurs in some patients with acute lymphoblastic leukaemia. The novel oncogene produces a tyrosine kinase, leading to cell proliferation.

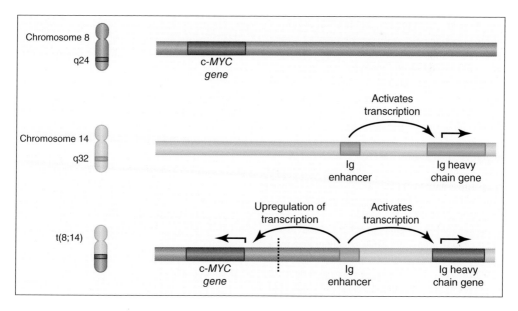

Figure 6.2 Upregulation of *c-MYC* in Burkitt lymphoma. A translocation between chromosome 14 and chromosome 8, t(8;14), juxtaposes the *c-MYC* oncogene with the immunoglobulin heavy chain gene enhancer, thereby upregulating the oncogene *c-MYC* and driving the cell into cycle. The translocation of an oncogene to the vicinity of the Ig gene regulatory elements is a common feature in B-cell lymphomas.

Classifying haematological malignancies: myeloid versus lymphoid disorders

As with all malignant disease, the cell of origin is of primary importance in classifying haematological malignancies. The most basic distinction is between myeloid and lymphoid malignancies, depending on the limb of the haematopoietic tree in which the malignancy arises and develops. This separation is used as a basis for the classification of haematological malignancies in this book. Within these two categories is a broad range of disease entities, with differing clinical and laboratory features.

Myeloid neoplasms – an introduction

Myeloid cells include the granulocytes (neutrophils, eosinophils, monocytes and basophils) and their precursors, as well as cells of the erythroid and megakaryocytic lineages. All of these arise from a multipotent common myeloid stem cell (see Chapter 1) which progressively differentiates and matures into lineage-specific effector cells under the influence of lineage-specific transcription factors. A neoplastic myeloid clone typically emerges relatively early in this process of myeloid maturation.

For the purposes of this text, we consider three main groups of malignant myeloid disorders: myeloproliferative neoplasms (MPNs), myelodysplastic syndromes (MDS) and acute myeloid leukaemia. The initial suspicion that a patient may have one of these disorders will come from abnormalities in the myeloid component of the blood count.

Acute myeloid leukaemia (AML) is a clonal disorder of myeloid progenitor cells characterized by a failure of myeloid maturation and rapid proliferation of immature blast cells. The diagnosis is made once myeloid blasts account for >20% of the nucleated cells seen on a bone marrow biopsy or blood smear (fewer blasts are needed for diagnosis where known pathogenic molecular changes have been identified). The failure of normal myeloid cell production means that patients tend to become rapidly unwell over a few weeks with symptoms of marrow failure (including breathlessness, infection and bleeding). It is recognized that there are several different subtypes of AML (typically classified by the genetic mutation present and/or morphological appearance). In *de novo* AML, there is no preceding history of a previous myeloid disorder (such as MDS or an MPN), nor previous exposure to cytotoxic and/or radiation therapy. Secondary AML arises from a preceding myeloid disorder or is due to previous chemotherapy or radiotherapy (where it is referred to as therapy-related AML or t-AML). Secondary AML tends to be more difficult to treat and cure than *de novo* AML.

The myelodysplastic syndromes are a heterogeneous group of disorders where the bone marrow is populated by an abnormal myeloid clone. These cells are dysplastic (i.e. look abnormal) and are often unable to mature normally, with fewer cells than normal emerging from the marrow into the blood. Patients therefore typically present with the symptoms of cytopenias, usually milder than those seen with AML but slowly progressive over time. The abnormal myeloid clone tends to accumulate further genetic mutations over time and in many cases leads to a more complete maturation block with blast accumulation, i.e. transformation to AML.

In the MPNs, there is increased proliferative activity within the myeloid lineage, though the affected cells retain their ability to mature and do not have significant functional defects. Four diseases are recognized in this category: polycythaemia vera (where red cell production is autonomously increased), chronic myeloid leukaemia (where granulocyte production is increased), essential thrombocythaemia (where too many platelets are generated) and primary myelofibrosis (where the marrow is replaced by fibrotic tissue due to abnormal haematopoeisis, particularly of the megakaryocyte lineage). The clinical presentation will vary depending on the cell type accumulating, but patients with MPNs may manifest problems with thrombosis, blood viscosity and splenomegaly (see also Chapter 8). As these are all clonal disorders, and may acquire further mutations, a proportion of patients will progress to develop acute myeloid leukaemia.

The myeloid disorders are explained in more detail in Chapter 8.

Lymphoid neoplasms – an introduction

Lymphomas are clonal malignant disorders that derive from lymphoid cells, either precursor or mature B or T cells. They are divided into two broad categories: Hodgkin lymphoma and non-Hodgkin lymphoma. Hodgkin lymphoma is diagnosed histologically by the presence of Reed–Sternberg cells within the appropriate cellular background. The non-Hodgkin lymphomas (NHL) are histologically heterogeneous and classified by their cell of origin – T, B or NK cells. The most common cell of origin by far is B cell. There are several different lymphomas and it is impractical for non-specialists to attempt to learn all subtypes. It is likely that within the current classification there will be additional entities not yet identified and refinement of subclassifications based upon immunophenotyping, cytogenetics and molecular analysis.

In clinical practice, non-Hodgkin lymphomas are sometimes divided into low and high grade (Table 6.2). Although this division is too imprecise to use as a definitive method for formal diagnosis, it still provides a useful framework for understanding these disorders. High-grade lymphomas are those that are rapidly fatal if left untreated, but can often be cured with multi-agent chemotherapy. They typically have a proliferative molecular basis (e.g. c-MYC dysregulation, as shown in Figure 6.2 above). Low-grade lymphomas generally have a low proliferation rate, and usually an anti-apoptotic molecular basis. They can be controlled with chemotherapy but are normally considered incurable with this treatment alone. Some low-grade lymphomas can be monitored for years without intervention. All low-grade lymphomas may transform into high-grade lymphoma, typically diffuse large B-cell lymphoma (DLCBL). The diseases of the lymphoid lineage are considered in more detail in chapter 9.

Plasma cell myeloma is a clonal disorder of plasma cells, one of the terminally differentiated cells of the B-lymphocyte lineage. It is considered separately from the lymphomas as it has different clinical features and is treated differently. Plasma cell myeloma is explained in more detail in Chapter 10.

Clinical manifestations

Many lymphoid malignancies will present with a palpable mass, in which case reaching the diagnosis is generally straightforward. However, some cases present diagnostic difficulties, since lymphomas are great mimickers of other diseases. Patients may present with constitutional symptoms of weight loss, fever or sweats (collectively termed B symptoms) and lymphoma is also a potential diagnosis in a patient with pyrexia of unknown origin. Pruritus is a further symptom that should prompt consideration of the diagnosis of lymphoma. Lymphomas may also present with obstructive symptoms, for example of the bowel, the bile duct (nodes in the porta hepatis) or the renal outflow tract. About 60% of lymphomas involve the lymph nodes; the remaining 40% can involve almost any organ of the body. The diagnosis is based on the histological appearances of an enlarged lymph node or other affected tissue or the cytology of blood or cerebrospinal fluid (CSF) in combination with immunophenotyping and immunohistochemistry (see also Chapter 7).

Leukaemias versus lymphomas

There is often confusion regarding the difference between leukaemias and lymphomas, and difficulties will arise if this (false) dichotomy is used to try and classify haematological malignancies. In thinking about haematological malignancies, the important question is always to determine the cell of origin. This is exactly how lymphomas are defined: all arise from lymphocytes or their precursors. The term *leukaemia* is not restricted to any cell of origin: it is, in many ways, a historical term and simply implies the presence of abnormal white cells in the blood or bone marrow. It follows, therefore, that some conditions (e.g. chronic lymphocytic leukaemia) can fit into both groups.

Rather than trying to classify haematological malignancies as leukaemias or lymphomas, it is more logical and simpler to classify them as lymphoid or myeloid in their origin. For example, lymphoblastic lymphoma and lymphoblastic leukaemia arise from the same cell of origin; their biology is identical and

Table 6.2 Examples of high- and low-grade lymphoid neoplasms.

Chronic lymphocytic leukaemia	Low grade
Follicular lymphoma	Low grade
Lymphoplasmacytic lymphoma	Low grade
Mantle cell lymphoma	Features of both low and high grade
Diffuse large B-cell lymphoma	High grade
Acute lymphoblastic leukaemia/ lymphoblastic lymphoma	High grade
Burkitt lymphoma	High grade

their treatment is also equivalent. Classifying one as a leukaemia and the other as a lymphoma is a biologically irrelevant distinction; classifying both by their cell of origin enhances understanding of the underlying disease and allows the delivery and development of rational treatments.

Premalignant clonal disorders in haematology

It is now well recognized that haematological malignancies are preceded by asymptomatic clonal disorders, which may be present for years preceding diagnosis. In the myeloid disorders myelodysplasia and AML, mutations in genes (most commonly *DNMT3A*, *TET2* and *ASXL1*) can be found several years prior to diagnosis in patients with normal blood counts. This is referred to as clonal haematopoeisis (CH). In chronic lymphocytic leukaemia, monoclonal B-cell lymphocytosis (a low-level lymphocytosis insufficient for a formal diagnosis of CLL, but nevertheless demonstrably clonal) can be detected for a number of years prior to diagnosis. Patients with plasma cell myeloma usually have a detectable paraprotein for several years prior to diagnosis – a condition referred to as monoclonal gammopathy of uncertain significance (MGUS).

All of these precursor conditions are common in the elderly (all being found at an incidence of 5–10% in the over-60s), and the challenge is therefore being able to predict if and when patients will develop a true symptomatic malignancy. As well as giving us valuable clues as to the multistep processes by which these diseases develop, such 'premalignant' conditions may also allow better care of patients at high risk and may even permit therapeutic interventions to delay or prevent development of symptomatic malignancy.

Staging of haematological malignancies

Staging is an important part of the initial clinical work-up of patients with *non-haematological* malignancies, highlighting the extend of spread of a primary tumour and defining which tissues are involved, with implications for the patient's prognosis. Since haematological malignancies affect, by definition, circulating cells, the concept of staging in these conditions is rather different.

Myeloid neoplasms are not formally staged at all. Disease present in one part of the bone marrow is deemed to be present in all bone marrow sites, and evidence of the clone can found in circulating blood cells too.

Staging in other haematological malignancies is performed for prognostic purposes, and not usually to define the extent of disease 'spread'; even apparently localized nodal involvement in lymphoma usually requires systemic treatment. The Ann Arbor staging system is used in lymphoma (Figure 6.3), with positron emission tomography/computed tomography (PET/CT) or CT scanning being the main modality for staging. Magnetic resonance imaging (MRI) is used for some sites, e.g. the central nervous system.

18F-Fluorodeoxyglucose (FDG)-PET in combination with CT imaging has become increasingly important in the management of lymphoma (Figure 6.4). It utilizes the observation that rapidly dividing malignant cells more readily take up glucose than non-malignant cells, and can demonstrate small foci of disease (in particular extranodal disease) which cannot be identified on CT scanning alone and may therefore 'upstage' disease and help guide appropriate treatment. Radiolabelled glucose is infused into the patient, and the tissues that take up the label may then be visualized by the PET scanner.

A separate 'staging' system is used for myeloma, using blood markers to give prognostic information, but again, the fluid nature of the malignancy means that disease is assumed to be widespread at diagnosis.

Assessment of disease status in this way is typically performed at diagnosis, and to gauge a patient's response to treatment; in myeloid diseases where radiological staging is not possible, reassessment of bone marrow morphology and (increasingly) molecular quantitation of residual disease are performed.

Principles of treatment for haematological malignancies

Treatment strategies for haematological malignancies need to take into account the nature of the disease

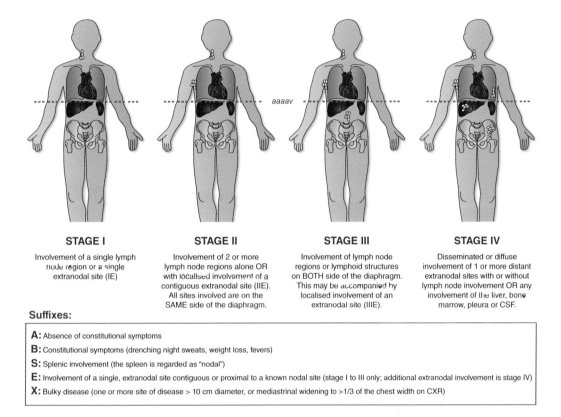

STAGE I	STAGE II	STAGE III	STAGE IV
Involvement of a single lymph node region or a single extranodal site (IE)	Involvement of 2 or more lymph node regions alone OR with localised involvement of a contiguous extranodal site (IIE). All sites involved are on the SAME side of the diaphragm.	Involvement of lymph node regions or lymphoid structures on BOTH side of the diaphragm. This may be accompanied by localised involvement of an extranodal site (IIIE).	Disseminated or diffuse involvement of 1 or more distant extranodal sites with or without lymph node involvement OR any involvement of the liver, bone marrow, pleura or CSF.

Suffixes:

A: Absence of constitutional symptoms

B: Constitutional symptoms (drenching night sweats, weight loss, fevers)

S: Splenic involvement (the spleen is regarded as "nodal")

E: Involvement of a single, extranodal site contiguous or proximal to a known nodal site (stage I to III only; additional extranodal involvement is stage IV)

X: Bulky disease (one or more site of disease > 10 cm diameter, or mediastrinal widening to >1/3 of the chest width on CXR)

Figure 6.3 The staging system used in both Hodgkin and non-Hodgkin lymphoma.
Source: Courtesy of Dr Caroline Watson.

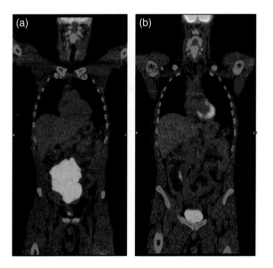

Figure 6.4 (a) A PET-CT showing relapsed DLBCL following an autologous stem cell transplant with a large intra-abdominal mass. (b) Following CAR T-cell therapy, the patient achieved a complete metabolic remission.
Source: Courtesy of Dr Iosif Mendichovszky, Cambridge University Hospitals NHS Foundation Trust.

(its aggressiveness and expected natural history), its known sensitivity to treatment agents, the general health status of the patient and their personal preferences.

Many haematological malignancies can be treated with curative intent, including many high-grade lymphomas (e.g. diffuse large B-cell lymphoma, Burkitt lymphoma). In these cases, aggressive combination chemotherapy is required. In other diseases, such as most low-grade lymphomas, standard cytotoxic chemotherapy cannot effect a cure, and treatment is therefore given when needed for symptomatic purposes. A 'watch and wait' approach (active surveillance) means that patients can be treated only as needed.

As we come to understand more of the molecular basis for haematological malignancies, therapies targeting the pathophysiology directly are becoming more widely available. From the initial example of imatinib in chronic myeloid leukaemia, we now see targeted 'chemotherapy-free' treatments for subtypes of AML and immunotherapies targeting specific anomalies seen in lymphomas. Although these targeted treatments may avoid some of the expected side-effects of conventional chemotherapy (nausea, vomiting, hair loss, infertility), they usually have a range of other adverse effects which need to be managed carefully to provide the best outcome for patients.

Good outcomes are also dependent on meticulous supportive care (Table 6.3). Most patients with a diagnosis of a haematological malignancy will have their case reviewed and discussed by a specialist multidisciplinary team, including haematologists, specialist radiologists and pathologists, specialist nurses and pharmacists.

Table 6.3 Supportive care.

Requirement	Comments
Venous access	Most patients will have a tunnelled line (Hickman line) inserted via the jugular or subclavian veins for ease of administration of chemotherapy and blood products. A peripherally inserted central catheter (PICC) may also be used
Blood product support	Many chemotherapy regimens suppress marrow function. Red cell and platelet support is likely to be needed. Transfusion thresholds are centre- and patient-specific. A typical transfusion threshold would be 80 g/L for haemoglobin and 10×10^9/L for platelets in the absence of bleeding or fever
Antiemetic therapy	Nausea and vomiting can be debilitating side-effects of conventional chemotherapy. Treatments include $5\text{-}HT_3$ antagonists such as ondansetron; dexamethasone, cyclizine, methoclopramide and NK1 receptor antagonists may all play a role
Fertility preservation	Sperm banking should be offered before cytotoxic chemotherapy, where practical. For women, specialist advice is needed; egg freezing may be possible depending upon urgency of chemotherapy
Nutritional support	Either via oral supplementation or total parenteral nutrition where food cannot be absorbed by the gut
Infection prophylaxis	Aciclovir used as prophylaxis against herpes simplex virus or varicella zoster virus reactivation. Ciprofloxacin may be used as prophylaxis against Gram-negative sepsis. Some patients may require antifungal prophylaxis. Granulocyte colony stimulating factor (G-CSF) shortens the duration of neutropenia and is often used, particularly during intensive treatments

7

Cellular and molecular investigations in haematology

LEARNING OBJECTIVES

After reading this chapter, you should be able to:

- ✔ describe the principles and uses of immunophenotyping by flow cytometry
- ✔ understand the role of karyotyping and fluorescence *in situ* hybridization (FISH) in the diagnosis and risk stratification of haematological malignancies
- ✔ describe the principle and utility of the polymerase chain reaction in diagnostics
- ✔ apply clonality studies in diagnosing lymphoproliferative diseases
- ✔ appreciate the significance of next-generation sequencing in diagnostics
- ✔ understand the importance of integrating clinical, morphological, cellular and molecular analyses in making haematological diagnoses.

While the blood count remains the key initial investigation in the diagnosis of most haematological diseases, our understanding of their molecular basis means that increasingly sophisticated cellular and molecular tests are used to diagnose, risk-stratify and monitor these conditions. Genetic analysis has been considered in passing when discussing the diagnosis of inherited haemolytic conditions and globin disorders (see Chapters 4 and 5) but molecular and genetic analysis is also central to the investigation and follow-up of patients with malignant haematological disease. To inform the discussion of these diseases in subsequent chapters, the key cellular, molecular and genetic investigations in general clinical use are outlined here.

Many of these techniques will be mentioned again in disease-specific contexts in the following chapters.

Immunophenotyping

Many cell types in the blood can be identified accurately simply by inspecting a peripheral blood film: neutrophils, eosinophils, basophils and monocytes are among these. While it is possible to identify lymphocytes morphologically, it is not possible to be confident about whether they are B cells or T cells. Similarly, although blasts can be identified in the

Haematology Lecture Notes, Eleventh Edition. Deborah Hay, Andrew King and Michael Desborough.
© 2023 John Wiley & Sons Ltd. Published 2023 by John Wiley & Sons Ltd.
Companion website: www.wiley.com/go/Hay/Haematology/11e

blood film by their large size, immature appearance and characteristic chromatin texture, it is not always possible to determine by inspection alone if they are of the myeloid or lymphoid lineage. These questions are of significance diagnostically and in determining treatment, and we rely on the technique of immunophenotyping by flow cytometry to answer them.

Immunophenotyping starts with the principle that specific antibodies can bind to individual markers ('cluster of differentiation' or CD markers) on the surface of blood cells. If these antibodies are conjugated to a fluorescent tag, it becomes possible to determine which cells in a population bear each cell surface marker; and using combinations of different fluorescent tags for different CD markers allows combinations of CD markers to be detected on individual cells. In this way, a population of abnormal lymphocytes in a blood sample may be defined as being either T cells (bearing CD3, for example, on their surface) or B cells (bearing CD20). Specific abnormal combinations of cell surface markers are also seen in specific diseases, such as chronic lymphocytic leukaemia (see also Chapter 9). This technique can also determine the clonality of lymphoid and plasma cell populations by examining expression of the κ versus λ immunoglobulin light chains. Likewise, a blast population identified in the blood can be shown to be either myeloid or lymphoid in origin on the basis of the CD markers they express.

Figure 7.1 gives a schematic representation of the process of flow cytometry. First, hydrodynamic

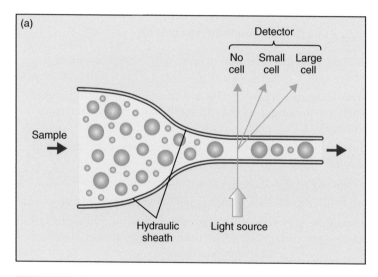

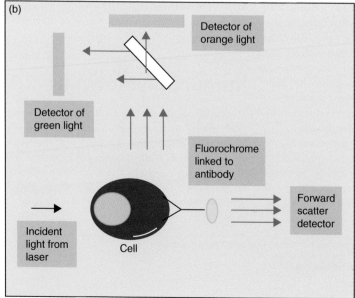

Figure 7.1 (a) Schematic diagram showing how cells are presented to a laser light beam by hydrodynamic focusing. (b) Schematic diagram to illustrate general principles of flow cytometry.

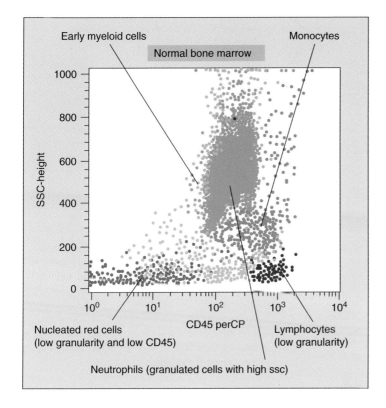

Figure 7.2 Flow cytometry of normal bone marrow after incubating normal bone marrow cells with PerCP-labelled anti-CD45 antibody. ssc, side scatter.

focusing is used to guide cells one by one through a narrow inlet in which they are exposed to a laser light source. The size of the cell will determine the degree of 'forward' scatter of the incident light as shown in panel (a); the degree of cellular complexity (e.g. the presence of a lobed nucleus or cytoplasmic granules) will also give 'side scatter' of the incident light, allowing differentiation of some cellular populations even without the need for specific fluorochromes.

When cells are incubated with fluorochrome-labelled antibodies before being subjected to the laser light, the colour of the light emitted by the fluorochrome will be detected if the cell being analysed bears the antigen in question. In panel (b), two wavelengths of light are detected, corresponding to the light emitted by the fluorochromes fluorescein isothiocyanate (FITC, green) and phycoerythrin (PE, orange). Multiparametric flow cytometry can assess many markers on an individual cell, and can assess many thousands of cells from a liquid sample (blood, liquid bone marrow aspirate, cerebrospinal fluid, pleural fluid, etc.) in minutes. Figure 7.2 shows a simple plot of side scatter (*y* axis) against expression of the common leucocyte antigen CD45, which allows separation of many of the cell types present in normal blood.

Cytogenetics and fluorescence *in situ* hybridization

Some diagnoses in haematology rely on the presence of a particular chromosomal translocation. The presence of t(9;22), the Philadelphia chromosome, in chronic myeloid leukaemia (see also Chapter 8) is perhaps the best known example, but many more exist with either diagnostic or prognostic significance (Table 7.1).

Cytogenetic analysis involves examination and identification of the full complement of chromosomes in the cell. Chromosomes are identified by their G-banding pattern, which represents the density of bases A and T versus G and C. The pattern of light and dark staining that results from the varying distribution of base pairs can be used to identify individual chromosomes and thus to give a complete karyotype (Figure 7.3).

Abnormalities in chromosome number (known as aneuploidy) include monosomy (loss of a single copy of one chromosome, e.g. monosomy 7 and monosomy 5 in both myelodysplasia and AML), trisomy (e.g. trisomy 8, also seen in some myeloid disorders) and

Table 7.1 Selected chromosomal translocations associated with haematological disease.

Translocation	Genes affected	Disease	Comments
t(8;12)	*AML1, ETO*	Acute myeloid leukaemia (AML)	Good prognostic feature in AML
t(8;14)	*c-MYC, IGH*	Burkitt lymphoma	Upregulation of *c-MYC* expression results from juxtaposition with *IGH* regulatory elements
t(9;22)	*BCR, ABL1*	Chronic myeloid leukaemia Also some cases of acute lymphoblastic leukaemia	Philadelphia chromosome; translocation encodes a constitutively active tyrosine kinase
t(11;14)	*CCND1, IGH*	Mantle cell lymphoma	Places the *CCND1* gene under the control of the *IGH* promoter
t(14;18)	*BCL2, IGH*	Follicular lymphoma	*BCL2* overexpression results from juxtaposition with *IGH* joining segment
t(15;17)	*PML, RAR1*	Acute promyelocytic leukaemia	Abnormal retinoic acid receptor created, blocking differentiation
Inv(16)	*MYH11, CBFB*	AML	Good prognostic feature in AML

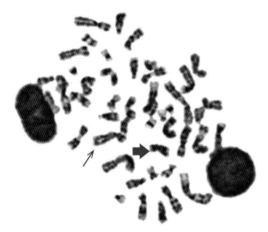

Figure 7.3 G-banded metaphase spread showing deletion of 5q. Thin arrow, normal chromosome 5; thick arrow, del(5q).
Source: Courtesy of Carolyn Campbell, Oxford University Hospitals.

hyperdiploidy (a good prognostic feature in childhood acute lymphoblastic leukaemia). Karyotypic analysis can also detect partial loss of chromosomes (e.g. del(5q), responsible for a specific, good prognostic subtype of myelodysplasia) and chromosomal translocations (such as the Philadelphia chromosome in chronic myeloid leukaemia).

In order to be able to see the characteristics of individual chromosomes and their banding patterns, the cells must be arrested in metaphase. To do this, dividing cells are harvested from the bone marrow and grown in culture for 24–48 hours before metaphase arrest is induced by the addition of an agent that prevents mitotic spindle formation.

Disruption of the cell membrane allows the creation of a metaphase spread, which is then organized into a karyotype for ease of interpretation.

Molecular cytogenetic techniques allow an additional level of detail in the analysis of structural chromosomal abnormalities. They rely on the binding of DNA or RNA probes to relevant complementary DNA sequences on a chromosome. Linking a fluorochrome to the probe means that regions of interest on a chromosome can be visualized by dark-field microscopy. This is fluorescence *in situ* hybridization (FISH).

Using FISH to define the location of a single sequence of interest in nuclear space means it is possible to detect small deletions or gene duplications that would be hard to see with simple karyotyping. Adding a fluorochrome of a different colour to bind to another gene or region of interest also enables the demonstration of translocations. Figure 7.4, for example, shows red and green FISH probes binding to the *BCR* (green) and *ABL* (red) genes. As these probes bind to separate chromosomes (chromosomes 22 and 9, respectively), they are separated in nuclear space. In the presence of the Philadelphia chromosome, the two probes are physically apposed, and the red and green fluorescent probes overlap to give a single yellow signal. This is an example of a 'fusion probe'.

Fusion probes are clearly useful only if we know both sequences that are involved in the generation of a fusion gene; in the case of CML, we know these are *BCR* and *ABL*. However, in many cases, the fusion

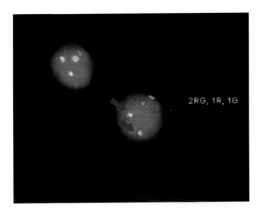

2RG, 1R, 1G

Figure 7.4 BCR/ABL1 FISH showing standard rearrangement consistent with t(9;22). Both cells shown have a single Philadelphia chromosome: the normal *BCR* and *ABL* signals are shown as the separate red and green signals; the two fused signals (arrowed in the lower cell) represent the derivative chromosomes each bearing part of the *BCR* gene and part of *ABL1*.
Source: Courtesy of Carolyn Campbell, Oxford University Hospitals.

Table 7.2 Selected genes frequently mutated in haematological disease.

Disease group	Genes bearing recurrent mutations
Myeloproliferative neoplasms	*JAK2, MPL, calreticulin*
Myelodysplasia and acute myeloid leukaemia	*NPM1, FLT3, IDH1 & 2, DNMT3, TET2, EZH2, ASXL1*
Chronic lymphocytic leukaemia	*TP53, ATM, SF3B1, NOTCH1*
Diffuse large B-cell lymphoma, follicular lymphoma	*CARD11, TP53, MLL2, CREBBP, MYOM2, TNFAIP3*
Lymphoplasmacytoid lymphoma	*MYD88*
Hairy cell leukaemia	*BRAF*
Myeloma	*KRAS, NRAS, TP53, BRFA, FAM46C*
Acute lymphoblastic leukaemia	*TP53, NRAS, KRAS, PAX5, JAK2, FLT3*

partners and their sequence/chromosomal location are not known, or there may be several potential fusion partners from which to choose. In this situation, 'break-apart' probes can be used. Here, differently coloured probes are hybridized to either end of a gene of interest. Normally, these probes will be closely apposed in nuclear space, and will give a single fused signal. However, if there is a translocation resulting in separation of the two ends of the gene, the two probes will be physically separated and thus give two distinct signals.

Fluorescence *in situ* hybridization is a demanding technique, and typically a sample of the order of 200 cells may be examined. This necessarily limits its sensitivity for the assessment of remission (see section on RT-PCR).

Molecular genetics

Karyotyping and FISH are unsuitable for the detection of fine-scale genetic changes such as point mutations or small insertions and deletions, yet mutations of this type are widely recognized as significant in the causation of haematological disease. Table 7.2 gives examples of genes in which mutations have been commonly identified in haematological disease. Molecular genetic analysis is required to detect these changes, and is an important part of the work of the modern haematology laboratory. Further, an appreciation of the signalling pathways most commonly disrupted is valuable in designing rational treatments.

Polymerase chain reaction

Polymerase chain reaction (PCR) is one of the most widely used techniques in molecular genetics. It is rapid, inexpensive and, providing stringent steps are taken to avoid sample contamination, highly reliable.

The technique is based on thermal cycling – that is, the sequential exposure of DNA to high and moderate temperatures in the presence of a heat-stable DNA polymerase and primers and nucleotides for the synthesis of further DNA strands. At high temperatures (>95 °C), the two complementary strands of DNA separate (denature). A cooler phase follows, in which short nucleotide sequences known as primers anneal to the two exposed DNA strands. These primers form the beginning of a new DNA strand, synthesized by the DNA polymerase using free nucleotides during a third phase (extension, typically at 72 °C), with the original DNA strand used as a template. This three-step process can be repeated many times, yielding exponential amplification of the amount of target DNA sequence (Figure 7.5).

The PCR product can be visualized on an agarose gel, and its size determined by comparison with markers of known molecular weight. Thus, deletions or duplications within the amplified sequence can be determined (see also section on clonality studies). If the primers used to generate the PCR product include nucleotides affected by known pathogenic mutations, the reaction can be designed to yield a product only when a known deletion is present. This is termed *allele-specific PCR* and has both good sensitivity and specificity for known mutations.

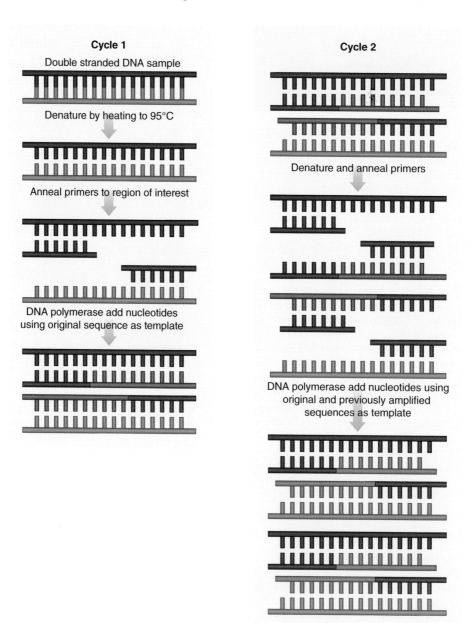

Figure 7.5 Schematic representation of the polymerase chain reaction (PCR). Here a single copy of double-stranded DNA is used as the starting template. Following two cycles of PCR, four copies are generated; an ongoing exponential increase is achieved with further cycles, and many millions of target copies will be generated by a standard PCR.

Clonality studies

Polymerase chain reaction also has a role in the investigation of clonality of lymphoid populations. A lymphocytosis in the peripheral blood may be reactive, as in viral conditions, or clonal as in B- and T-cell lymphoproliferative disorders. While immunophenotyping may be able to define B-cell clonality through the expression of either the κ or λ light chain of the immunoglobulin molecule, there is no widely available similar simple immunophenotypic test to determine clonality in populations of T cells.

The T-cell receptor (TCR) gene locus undergoes rearrangement (known as VDJ recombination; see also Chapter 1) during maturation of the T cell, leading to a vast repertoire of TCR specificities. In the context of clonal lymphocytosis, the TCR will be of only a single specificity; in a reactive lymphocytosis, the selection of T cells responding to a variety of antigenic epitopes means that TCRs of several specificities will be generated. This difference between clonal and polyclonal T-cell populations can be exploited for diagnostic purposes.

T-cell clonality studies use PCR as described above, multiplexed with primers designed to capture the most widely used VDJ domains. The amplified DNA fragments will be of varying sizes in the context of a polyclonal population, and many peaks will be visualized when the fragment sizes are quantified by GeneScan® analysis. By contrast, a clonal population will give a single TCR amplification product, and thus a single peak (or very restricted profile) when the fragment sizes are assessed (Figure 7.6). A similar process can be used to assess the immunoglobulin gene rearrangement in B-cell populations to assess clonality and to give prognostic information in some lymphoproliferative conditions.

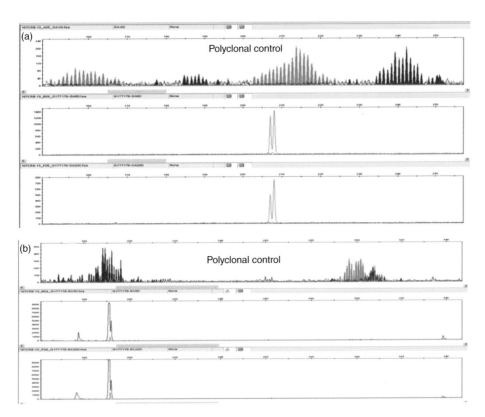

Figure 7.6 Two GeneScan plots showing the results of clonality assessment at the *TCRG* locus (a) and *TCRB* locus (b). In each panel, the top trace shows a polyclonal control with a range of PCR product sizes; the lower two traces in each panel are consistent with a monoclonal pattern of TCR rearrangement. Performed using BIOMED2 primers. The *y*-axis denotes the amount of PCR product; the *x*-axis shows the size of the PCR product.

Useful though clonality studies may be, their interpretation is not without pitfalls. Elderly patients may naturally have a more oligoclonal pattern than younger individuals, and a severely oligoclonal or even monoclonal pattern may be seen as part of the reactive immune response to a dominant antigen. This 'pseudoclonality' has the potential to be misleading, and it is vital that clonality studies are interpreted only in the complete clinical context if they are to give useful diagnostic information.

Real-time or semiquantitative PCR

The techniques described above will allow laboratory haematologists to determine whether or not a specific mutation or rearrangement is present. They do not describe the degree of expression of abnormal genes, nor can they give sensitive information regarding the relative size of a malignant clone of cells. In order to do this, gene expression is assessed in addition to gene sequence.

Reverse transcription PCR (RT-PCR, also known as real-time PCR or semiquantitative PCR, qPCR) permits this. With this technique, RNA is isolated from the sample of interest and reverse-transcribed to produce cDNA. This is then the subject of PCR amplification which can be monitored in real time. By including a fluorescent probe to the target sequence which is released during the amplification phase, the amount of a specific cDNA sequence in a sample can be assessed, and contrasted with a stable control cDNA sequence. The technique can therefore give a measure of the number of transcripts of a given gene relative to a control gene.

For conditions in which a known abnormal transcript is produced (e.g. the BCR-ABL1 fusion transcript in chronic myeloid leukaemia (CML), or the PML-RARA fusion transcript in acute promyelocytic leukaemia; see also Chapter 8), RT-PCR is a powerful technique for assessing whether ongoing transcription is occurring. The depth of remission can therefore be assessed at a molecular level, far more sensitively than would be possible with either morphological assessment of the blood or marrow or FISH analysis of a limited number of cells. It is therefore widely used for disease monitoring and the detection of measurable residual disease where an appropriate disease-specific transcript is available (Figure 7.7).

Next-generation sequencing

The techniques described above focus on the investigation of a single suspected mutation or chromosomal translocation. It is becoming clear, however, that the molecular genetic landscape of many malignancies is much more complex. Multiple clones may exist in a given sample, with many mutations; some may be true 'driver' mutations responsible for the

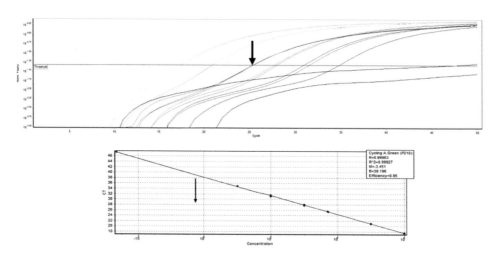

Figure 7.7 Relative quantitation of abnormal transcript levels by quantitative PCR (qPCR). The top panel shows a qPCR trace in which five dilutions of a known concentration control transcript (turquoise to dark blue) have been run alongside a patient sample (green). The amount of transcript relative to the standard can then be read from a standard curve (lower panel).

de novo development of malignant change, while others arise as a consequence of the genetic instability induced by earlier mutations. Unravelling the clinical significance of such complex genetic changes is a major challenge for all clinicians involved in the care of patients with haematological malignancies.

The gold standard technique for sequencing DNA remains Sanger sequencing. This technique starts with PCR to amplify the region of interest. The PCR product is then subject to further rounds of amplification with modified nucleotides that feature a fluorescently labelled 'terminator' added to the reaction mix. A different fluorescent marker is used for each of the four different terminator nucleotides, which, when incorporated into the PCR product, prevent the addition of any further nucleotides. The result is a mix of PCR products of varying lengths, each ending with a fluorescent label, the colour of which depends on the final nucleotide incorporated. This permits the original DNA sequence to be deduced (Figure 7.8).

Clearly, this technique can be employed only for relatively short sequences and limited numbers of targets. Next-generation sequencing (NGS), by contrast, can rapidly produce data for many target sequences. The process of NGS is summarized schematically in Figure 7.9. Here, DNA from a patient sample is sheared either physically or enzymatically into short fragments. Oligonucleotide linkers are then attached to the ends of the DNA fragments. This 'library' of DNA fragments is then supported on a microscope slide to which oligonucleotides complementary to those flanking the DNA fragments are attached. Thus, the DNA library is attached to a solid platform for all downstream steps.

The immobilized DNA library is then subject to PCR amplification to create clusters in which identical DNA fragments are colocated on the slide. From here, the process of Sanger sequencing is performed, with the additional benefit of spatial imaging: each immobilized DNA cluster on the slide can be directly imaged, and the consequence of incorporating a fluorescently labelled terminator nucleotide can be recorded. The imaging phase is followed by a wash-out phase, in which the terminator nucleotide is repaired to remove the fluorescent label and permit further extension of the DNA. The cycle can then be repeated to determine the next nucleotide in sequence, not for one DNA molecule or one amplified cluster, but for hundreds of thousands of clusters simultaneously. The sequential incorporation of each nucleotide, manifest by a specific fluorescent signal at each DNA cluster, is detected and recorded by sequencing software, and the overall sequence for each DNA cluster is determined computationally. This massively parallel approach makes it possible to determine extended sequences in a short timeframe. Reconstruction of the sequence data collected against the reference genome requires careful bioinformatic analysis.

Many variations on this theme exist with different sequencing techniques and varying methodologies. However, all have in common the capacity to achieve high-fidelity extended DNA sequences in a relatively short timeframe. This has been extended to whole exomes and even whole genomes, but is currently most widely used in the clinical setting for the interrogation of a number of known relevant gene targets.

Targeted resequencing panels use NGS to assess the sequence of several hundred genes (or mutation hotspots within genes) to provide a detailed genetic analysis of a given sample, without recourse to the expense or complexity of whole-genome or whole-exome sequencing.

An integrated haematology laboratory report

Integration of data from a range of laboratory modalities is essential if comprehensive diagnostic and prognostic information is to be delivered to clinicians treating patients with haematological disease. Many specialist haematology laboratories now produce a single integrated report which includes histopathology and cytology reports alongside blood counts and detailed molecular analysis. This is then used alongside clinical and radiological correlation to determine a final diagnosis.

Personalized medicine and redefining disease

Molecular genetic techniques have the potential to yield vast amounts of information concerning sequence variants throughout patient genomes, and we are now able to generate far more data than we are confidently able to interpret in the clinical setting. Major translational research programmes are therefore aiming to integrate extensive genomic

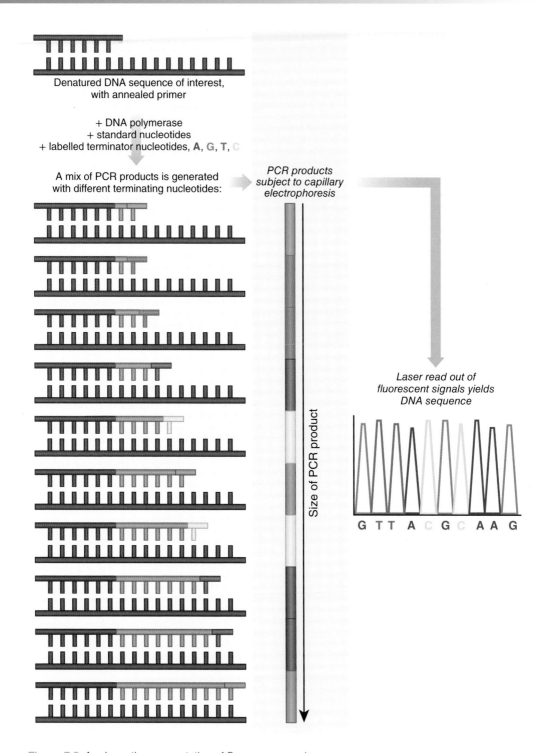

Figure 7.8 A schematic representation of Sanger sequencing.

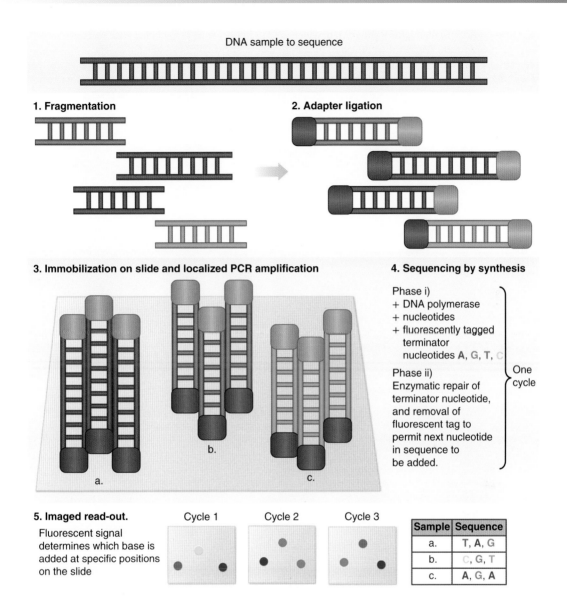

Figure 7.9 An overview of next-generation sequencing. See text for details.

datasets with clinical phenotypes and treatment outcomes in many different diseases. The UK's '100 000 Genomes' project is one such programme, and it is hoped that this will provide a step towards medicine that is truly personalized at the level of the patient's genome.

Moreover, the interface of laboratory genetic analysis and clinical haematology is leading to a need to define new disease entities. Where a patient is found to have a mutation in a gene recurrently affected in myelodysplasia, for example (see also Chapter 8), but does not meet formal diagnostic criteria for this disorder, how should the patient and their doctor respond to the presence of the mutation? The concept of 'clonal haematopoiesis of indeterminate potential', or CHIP, has arisen to describe this situation, and has opened new avenues for investigation of the mechanisms by which malignant diseases of the myeloid lineages arise. Likewise, the term 'clonal cytopenias of uncertain significance' (CCUS) highlights a situation in which low blood counts are seen in the content of plausible causative mutations, but without the required morphological features needed to diagnose specific myeloid malignancies.

In future, we anticipate that such recurrent molecular changes will have greater weight in the formal diagnostic criteria for haematological disease. For now, they provide powerful supportive evidence and frequently suggest targets for treatment.

Neoplastic disorders of myeloid cells

The myeloid neoplasms, introduced in Chapter 6, include conditions in which there is a failure of maturation of the myeloid limb of haematopoiesis, as well as conditions in which there is uncontrolled overproduction of myeloid cells. Although relatively uncommon malignancies, they include some which present as genuine medical emergencies. Our growing understanding of the molecular basis of these conditions is slowly being translated into improved outcomes for patients.

Acute myeloid leukaemia

Acute myeloid leukaemia (AML) is a clonal disorder of myeloid progenitor cells that may occur in patients of any age, but becomes increasingly common in older people. It is the most common form of acute leukaemia in adults. By definition, acute leukaemia is the accumulation of immature blast cells in the bone marrow, such that they typically exceed 20% of the total cellularity. The failure of myeloid maturation means that normal production of red cells, neutrophils and platelets is prevented and the blasts cells which accumulate in the marrow may spill out into the blood – a highly abnormal clinical finding (Figure 8.1).

Symptoms and signs

The clinical features reflect the consequences of bone marrow failure. Anaemia causes pallor, tiredness and exertional dyspnoea; neutropenia leads to infection, which may be life-threatening; and thrombocytopenia causes bleeding, bruising and purpura. Any patient presenting with such features requires urgent haematological assessment. Blast cells may infiltrate other organs such as the skin or gums (particularly in

Haematology Lecture Notes, Eleventh Edition. Deborah Hay, Andrew King and Michael Desborough.
© 2023 John Wiley & Sons Ltd. Published 2023 by John Wiley & Sons Ltd.
Companion website: www.wiley.com/go/Hay/Haematology/11e

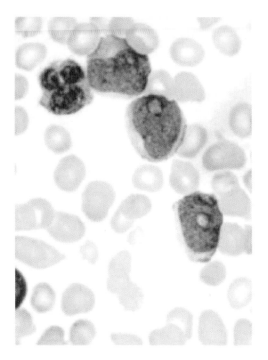

Figure 8.1 Acute myeloid leukaemia. The three leukaemic myeloblasts are considerably larger than adjacent red cells, have finely stippled nuclear chromatin and show prominent nucleoli. May–Grünwald–Giemsa (MGG) stain.

Any patient with unexplained pancytopenia or blast cells in the peripheral blood will require further investigation, and this will usually involve a bone marrow biopsy. Formal diagnosis of AML requires the bone marrow to contain >20% blast cells (with the exception of some cases in which disease-causing chromosomal translocations are identified), and blasts sometimes account for the overwhelming majority of nucleated cells seen.

Acute myeloid leukaemia must be distinguished from acute lymphoblastic leukaemia (ALL), another disorder in which the marrow is heavily infiltrated with blasts. This is important because their treatment and management differ significantly. Inspection of blasts morphologically on a bone marrow or blood film usually provides the likely diagnosis; for example, the presence of Auer rods, thin cytoplasmic inclusions formed by fusion of granules within blast cells, nearly always indicates AML (Figure 8.2). However, immunophenotyping using flow cytometry will usually be

cases where the blasts have an element of monocytic differentiation), and there may occasionally be lymphadenopathy and splenomegaly. Massive splenomegaly is unusual in this disorder, however. Blast cells can invade the central nervous system (CNS), although this is more common at relapse. There is also a higher incidence of CNS infiltration in paediatric cases.

Laboratory findings

The laboratory findings, like the clinical findings, reflect bone marrow failure. Anaemia results from inadequate red cell production. Thrombocytopenia is nearly always present and results both from a failure of production and from increased consumption. Some cases of AML, in particular acute promyelocytic leukaemia (APL), are associated with disseminated intravascular coagulation with abnormalities of haemostasis (see below). While neutropenia is almost always seen, the total white cell count (WCC) will be high in around half of all cases, reflecting a circulating population of blasts.

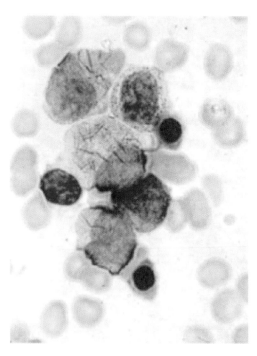

Figure 8.2 Myeloblasts of AML showing several Auer rods (MGG stain). These are azurophilic rod-shaped cytoplasmic inclusions that are exclusively found in some of the leukaemic myeloblasts of a small proportion of patients with AML, or chronic myeloid leukaemia (CML) in blast cell transformation.

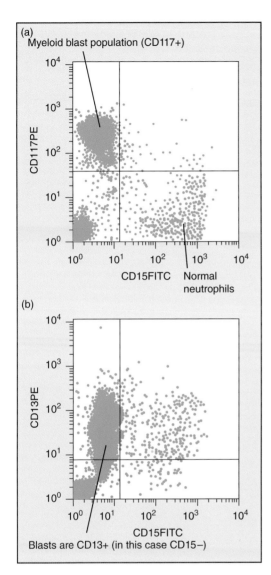

(a) Myeloid blast population (CD117+)

CD117PE

CD15FITC   Normal neutrophils

(b)

CD13PE

CD15FITC

Blasts are CD13+ (in this case CD15−)

Figure 8.3 Flow cytometry demonstrating myeloid antigen expression in a case of AML. The blasts are CD117+ and CD13+.

to provide genetic markers for measuring low-level residual disease following treatment (Box 8.1).

How does AML arise?

It is now recognised that AML is preceded by the precursor condition clonal haematopoeisis (CH). In CH, mutations in particular genes can be demonstrated prior to the development of abnormal blood counts or symptoms, indicating the presence of expanded myeloid clones. The most commonly mutated genes are *DNTM3A*, *TET2* and *ASXL1*, all genes implicated in epigenetic transcriptional regulation. CH is common, being found in 10% of patients over 60. The risk of developing a significant myeloid neoplasm such as myelodysplasia or AML is around 0.5-1% a year, and the majority of patients therefore never develop a

performed (Figure 8.3), showing myeloid antigens such as CD13, CD15, CD33, as well as the stem cell marker CD34 and stem cell factor receptor c-kit (CD117).

Genetic abnormalities are now also sought in all cases of AML, including both cytogenetic changes and mutations in genes recurrently mutated in myeloid disease. These are useful both prognostically and symptomatic disorder. Strategies for understanding the risk posed by specific mutations will therefore be important to be able to counsel patients effectively when CH is diagnosed.

DNA damage induced by radiation and previous chemotherapy exposure also increases the risk of AML. There are rare instances when individuals have a predisposition to AML; for example, children affected with Down syndrome have a 400 times higher incidence of a specific subtype of leukaemia compared with unaffected children, and some bone marrow failure syndromes (see Chapter 11) are associated with the development of acute leukaemia. Rarely, some families have inherited mutations of critical haematopoietic proteins (e.g. *GATA2, CEBPA, DDX41*) that may give rise to AML.

Classification

The classification of AML is complex and has been subject to numerous revisions as our understanding of this disorder has grown. Initially, AML was classified simply by the appearance of blasts on light microscopy (i.e. describing the degree of maturation or differentiation evident morphologically). This has been progressively superseded by classifications which take account of recurrent genetic abnormalities and/or preceding treatment; these relate to the natural history of the disease in a more meaningful fashion. An overview of this classification is shown in Table 8.1.

Acute promyelocyte leukaemia–AML with t(15;17)(q22;q12); *PML-RARA*

One subtype of AML is worthy of special mention as a consequence of its challenging clinical presentation and targeted treatment approach. Acute promyelocytic leukaemia (APL) lies within the classification group of AML with recurrent genetic abnormalities, since it is characterized by a specific translocation, t(15;17)(q22;q12). The breakpoint on chromosome 17 falls within the gene for the retinoic acid receptor (RARα), which is normally needed for appropriate differentiation of the cell. The breakpoint on chromosome 15 falls within the gene known as *PML*, a nuclear regulatory factor needed to control the induction of apoptosis of the cell. As a result of the translocation, a new fusion gene called *PML-RARA* is produced; this encodes a DNA-binding protein, causing a maturation block.

This maturation block means that APL is characterized by the accumulation of promyelocytes, early

Table 8.1 Acute myeloid leukaemia (AML) classification.

AML subtype	Comments
AML with recurrent genetic abnormalities	Includes the good prognosis 'core-binding factor' AMLs with known specific translocations, such as t(15;17) in acute promyelocytic leukaemia, amongst others with poorer prognosis. As the genetic change defines the disease, this does not always need >20% blasts
AML with myelodysplasia-related change (AML-MRC)	Requires a preceding history of myelodysplasia OR cytogenetic abnormalities associated with myelodysplasia, e.g. complex karyotype with 3 or more abnormalities, −7/del(7q), or del(5q)/t(5q) or evidence of dysplasia morphologically. Often poor prognosis. *TP53* mutations seen in ~1/3 of cases
Therapy-related myeloid neoplasm (t-AML)	In patients previously treated with drugs such as etoposide, alkylating agents or radiotherapy. Often multiple cytogenetic abnormalities, a high incidence of mutations in *TP53*, and a generally poor prognosis
AML, not otherwise specified	Approximately 30% of cases do not fit the categories above; a morphological classification based on blast morphology is used (e.g. AML without maturation, acute myelomonocytic leukemia, pure erythroid leukaemia)

granulocyte precursors with contain abundant granules and numerous Auer rods (Figure 8.4). Release of the promyelocytes' granules, which may occur spontaneously or at the initiation of cytotoxic therapy, is known to produce uncontrolled activation of the clotting and fibrinolytic system (see Chapter 13). The result is disseminated intravascular coagulation (DIC) and potentially life-threatening bleeding.

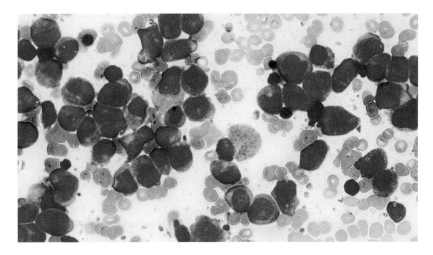

Figure 8.4 Bone marrow aspirate from a patient with acute promyelocytic leukaemia. The smear shows abundant, heavily granulated blasts, with occasional cells also having a classic bilobed nuclear morphology. Similar cells would be expected in the peripheral blood. MGG stain, ×40 magnification.

Treatment is with all-*trans* retinoic acid (ATRA) which binds the mutant PML-RARA protein and induces differentiation of the abnormal promyelocytes. This also limits the threat of DIC. Since the most dangerous period for patients with APL is shortly after diagnosis (when patients may have a significant coagulopathy, and are at risk of life-threatening haemorrhage and thrombosis), ATRA should be started without delay if APL is suspected, and coagulation parameters should be corrected.

After beginning treatment, patients may develop a differentiation syndrome, whereby an excessive inflammatory response occurs as leukaemic blasts differentiate. This manifests as weight gain due to fluid overload, fever, respiratory distress, acute kidney injury and a rising white cell count; it can be life-threatening. The risk is higher for those with a starting WCC >10 × 10^9/L. Differentiation syndrome is treated with high-dose dexamethasone and temporary cessation of leukaemia treatment.

After the first 2 weeks of treatment, the prognosis is excellent with the majority of patients being cured, now using a 'chemotherapy-free' approach which combines ATRA with another agent, arsenic trioxide (ATO). Monitoring for PML-RARA transcripts serves as an MRD marker and is performed to assess response to treatment.

Treatment of AML other than APL

Intensive treatment

The treatment given for AML depends upon the subtype, molecular mutations, age of the patient and comorbidities. Patients fit for curative treatment (typically those under the age of 70) are treated with intensive chemotherapy to try and obtain a remission (defined as a lack of morphological evidence of leukaemia on a bone marrow biopsy), which is then consolidated with further rounds of chemotherapy or an allogeneic stem cell transplant (see also Chapter 12), dependent upon the risk of relapse.

The backbone of intensive chemotherapy has remained the same for more than 30 years, and consists of an anthracycline (daunorubicin, D) given in combination with cytarabine (also known as Ara-C), a combination referred to as DA. Induction chemotherapy typically lasts 7–10 days, followed by a period of marrow aplasia for a further 3 weeks, before the normal bone marrow recovers. Patients are profoundly neutropenic and at risk of infection, including atypical infections such as fungal infections. They also require platelet and red cell transfusions. Inpatient admission is required for 4–5 weeks. Side-effects include cardiotoxicity, hair loss and mucositis.

More recently, a number of other agents have become available which are used as part of induction chemotherapy regimens (Table 8.2).

Induction therapy drug	Target	Comments
Gemtuzumab ozogamicin	CD33-targeting antibody with cytotoxic conjugate	Given with DA, improves outcomes in some AML subtypes. Requires CD33 expression
Midostaurin, gilteritinib	FLT3 inhibitors	Improved survival in patients with FLT3-mutated AML; utility in relapsed/refractory disease
CPX351	Liposomal formulation of cytarabine and daunorubicin	Particular efficacy in the AML-MRC and tAML categories. Most patients can avoid hair loss
Ivosidenib, enasidenib	IDH1 and IDH2 inhibitors	Target mutated IDH isoforms seen in some subtypes of AML

MRC, myelodysplasia-related change; tAML, therapy-related acute myeloid leukaemia.

Bone marrow transplantation (BMT)

For patients whose disease is considered to be high risk for relapse, allogeneic stem cell transplant offers a better chance of cure (see Chapter 12). Allogeneic BMT relies on using chemotherapy to reduce the leukaemia cell burden followed by infusion of donor stem cells. The donor marrow can then induce a 'graft versus leukaemia' effect, an immunological effect that eradicates chemoresistant disease. Conditioning chemotherapy may be myeloablative (i.e. high dose which ablates the bone marrow) or reduced intensity conditioning (lower dose where autologous haematopoietic recovery would normally occur). Myeloablative conditioning is normally used in younger patients (up to the age of 45); reduced intensity conditioning can be used in fit patients up to the age of 75.

Broadly, an allogeneic stem cell transplant halves the risk of relapse, but this has to be balanced against the considerable short-term and longer-term toxicity with a transplant-related mortality of 15–20%. It is therefore normally reserved for patients who have a >50% chance of relapse.

Non-intensive treatment

Patients deemed unfit for intensive chemotherapy have historically been offered supportive care (including antibiotics and blood transfusions), low-dose cytarabine or hypomethylating agents such as azacytidine or decitabine. Newer agents such as venetoclax, which promotes programmed cell death, are now routinely being used alongside other therapies, though outcomes remain poor.

Relapsed/refractory patients

Patients who are refractory or relapse after completing chemotherapy may be treated with further intensive chemotherapy (typically fludarabine, high-dose cytarabine and idarubicin administered with GCSF – FLAG-IDA) and then undergo an allogeneic stem cell transplant, assuming they achieve an adequate response. For those who do not achieve a sustained remission, good supportive care is critical.

Prognosis

The prognosis strongly depends upon the subtype of AML, genetic profile and therapy offered. APL is cured in the majority of cases (>95%) with ATO/ATRA. Some favourable risk subtypes of AML have cure rates of 70–80% (for example, t(8;21) and inv(16)). By contrast, complex karyotype *TP53* mutated AML has a cure rate at best of 10–20% even with intensive chemotherapy and an allogeneic stem cell transplant. Treatment for elderly patients with AML remains a significant challenge, with most patients dying within 2 years; newer agents show promise of significant improvements in overall survival.

Myelodysplastic syndromes

The myelodysplastic syndromes (MDS) are a collection of serious, relatively common disorders in which the bone marrow is populated by a clone of abnormal haematopoietic cells. Myeloid maturation is functionally abnormal and morphologically dysplastic (Figure 8.5), leading to peripheral blood cytopenias and their clinical consequences of anaemia, infection and bruising/bleeding. However, the clinical picture tends to be more indolent and slowly progressive

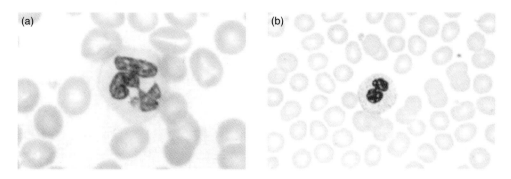

Figure 8.5 (a) Hypogranular neutrophil from a patient with myelodysplastic syndrome. Note the lack of granules in the cytoplasm. (b) Neutrophil granulocyte from a heterozygote for the inherited Pelger–Huet anomaly. The nucleus is bilobed (spectacle-like) and has markedly condensed chromatin. In heterozygotes for this asymptomatic condition, 50–70% of neutrophils show these changes. Similar abnormalities may be found in some neutrophils, as an acquired condition in MDS.

than that seen in AML where there is a complete maturation block.

The clinical and blood count features of MDS tend to worsen over time, with the acquisition of additional genetic aberrations. This leads to an accumulation of blast cells and ultimately the disorder may lead to bone marrow failure, either as a result of a transformation to acute leukaemia or because of stem cell failure. The marrow blast count, severity of cytopenias and underlying genetic abnormalities determine the prognosis.

The disease is most common in the elderly and is rare before the age of 50 years. MDS presents most commonly with symptoms of anaemia, but infection, bruising or bleeding may also occur. MDS has been subdivided into a number of categories depending on the presence of underlying cytogenetic abnormalities and morphological features such as ring sideroblasts. Patients may develop therapy-related MDS, secondary to chemotherapy and/or radiotherapy for other malignancies.

Typically, there is reduction in at least two cell lines (e.g. anaemia and neutropenia, or anaemia and thrombocytopenia). The anaemia is frequently macrocytic (not resulting from vitamin B12 or folate deficiency) and the neutrophils are 'dysplastic' – they look bizarre, often with reduced granulation and abnormal nuclear maturation, including the characteristic bilobed spectacle-like nuclei (Figure 8.5). Blasts cells may be found in low numbers in the peripheral blood. An increase in peripheral blood monocytes ($>1 \times 10^9$/L) defines these patients as having chronic myelomonocytic leukaemia (CMML), an unusual condition which has features of both a myeloproliferative disorder and myelodysplastic disorder and is therefore classed as an overlap MDS/MPN disorder. Cytogenetic abnormalities occur in about 50% of MDS cases, and key recurrent mutations in genes important for myeloid function are normally identified in cytogenetically normal cases and help confirm the diagnosis (Box 8.2).

Treatment

For patients with low-risk MDS, treatment is supportive. Erythropoietin may improve anaemia, and is sometimes combined with G-CSF in certain subtypes, where it may show synergy. Transfusion support with red cells and platelets may be necessary. Iron chelation is normally considered in patients receiving >20 red cell units. Thrombopoietin agonists such as eltrombopag and romiplostim may be given to thrombocytopenic patients to reduce the risk of bleeding.

For patients with intermediate- and high-risk MDS, hypomethylating agents including azacytidine and decitabine have been demonstrated to improve blood counts, thereby improving quality of life and ultimately survival (typically extending survival by approximately a year). These are given on an outpatient basis and are normally well tolerated, although cytopenias may worsen during the first 1–3 months of treatment.

For specific subtypes of MDS, specific treatments exist. Lenalidomide extends survival in MDS with the specific cytogenetic abnormality (del(5q). Luspatercept, which binds transforming growth factor-β superfamily ligands to reduce SMAD signalling (and therefore increases erythroid maturation) is used in

MDS with ring sideroblasts in order to reduce transfusion requirements. As our understanding of the pathogenesis of different subtypes of MDS expands, more targeted therapies are likely to become available.

Currently, the only curative strategy for myelodysplasia is allogeneic stem cell transplantation. This should be considered in all fit patients with MDS when the prognosis is less than ~3 years. The use of reduced intensity conditioning has expanded the possible age range up to 70–75 years.

Prognosis

The prognosis of MDS is variable, and depends on factors including the cytogenetic abnormalities, the genetic mutations, the bone marrow blast percentage and the degree and number of cytopenias. Patients may live as long as 15–20 years, or may only survive a few months. Adverse risk factors include a complex karyotype (where ≥3 cytogenetic abnormalities are present), a blast percentage of 10–19%, transfusion dependence and some genetic mutations such as *TP53*.

Myeloproliferative neoplasms

The myeloproliferative neoplasms (MPNs) are a group of diseases in which there is increased proliferative activity in one or more elements of the myeloid series, but with relatively normal maturation and little functional defect, unlike AML or MDS. The myeloproliferative neoplasms are chronic myeloid leukaemia (CML), polycythaemia vera, myelofibrosis and essential thrombocythaemia.

Chronic myeloid leukaemia

This condition, caused by the well-described chromosomal translocation t(9;22), is characterized by a massive proliferation of mature and maturing myeloid cells, particularly granulocytes. CML is very rare in children but increases in incidence with age. The symptoms are often vague and of insidious onset, and include constitutional symptoms such as fatigue, weight loss, sweats and anorexia. There may be few physical signs, but patients may be pale as a result of anaemia (the marrow space is almost exclusively taken over by the expanding granulocytic series), and there may be splenomegaly. Occasionally, patients with CML may present with symptoms of hyperviscosity because of a very high white cell count. Priapism, tinnitus and stupor are among the more common symptoms of this presentation.

Laboratory features

The peripheral blood abnormalities are characteristic. Patients are almost always anaemic and have elevated granulocyte counts (usually between 50 and 400×10^9/L), with excess neutrophils, myelocytes, metamyelocytes and basophils present in the peripheral blood (Figure 8.6); blast cells are also present but in small numbers (usually <10%). The bone marrow is very hypercellular, with greatly increased granulocyte production and increased numbers of megakaryocytes. Cytogenetic and molecular analysis is critical (see section on Philadelphia chromosome below).

Philadelphia chromosome

Chronic myeloid leukaemia is associated with a pathognomonic chromosomal rearrangement in which there is a reciprocal translocation between chromosomes 22 and 9. In this translocation, 5′ exons of *BCR* are fused to the 3′ exons of *ABL1*. This leads to the formation of a novel fusion gene that is transcribed into an oncoprotein with tyrosine kinase activity (BCR-ABL; Figure 8.7a); this is 210 kDa in size. This protein leads to increased cell cycling and a failure of apoptosis, with the accumulation of myeloid cells. The fusion chromosome 22q (with additional material from chromosome 9) is known as the *Philadelphia chromosome*.

The Ph translocation is also seen in acute lymphoblastic leukaemia. In some of these cases, the breakpoint in *BCR* is the same as that seen in CML; in others, however, the breakpoint is further upstream in the intron between the first and second exons, leaving only the first exon of *BCR* intact. This fusion protein is smaller, measuring 190 kDa.

The tyrosine kinase (TK) *BCR-ABL* is therefore an excellent target for therapy. Inhibitors of the ATP-binding site on this tyrosine kinase are used to treat CML. The first such compound that emerged as a specific inhibitor of BCR-ABL was imatinib, a generally well-tolerated oral agent that when taken daily can control the disease effectively, normally indefinitely (Figure 8.7b). Patients who are intolerant of imatinib or fail to respond can be treated with one of the newer tyrosine kinase inhibitors (TKIs) such as dasatinib or nilotinib. By blocking the inactive conformation of the BCR-ABL oncoprotein, TKIs allow inhibition of its oncogenetic activity and thereby treat CML at the molecular level.

Clinical course and treatment

The disorder runs a predictable course. In the first phase (*chronic phase*), normal blood counts are achieved with TKI therapy such as imatinib, and the patient is generally well. This phase may continue for many years. The disease may then transform through an *accelerated phase* (where blood counts become difficult to control) into *blast crisis*. This latter phase is defined by an increasing number of blasts in the bone

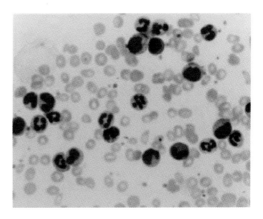

Figure 8.6 Blood film from a patient with CML showing an increased number of white cells, mainly neutrophils, band cells and metamyelocytes. Note the presence of some myelocytes and basophils.

marrow, and in terms of its natural history is akin to acute leukaemia. Symptomatically, patients describe weight loss, night sweats and fevers.

Switching to second- or third-line TKIs may be helpful when molecular monitoring of *BCR-ABL* transcript levels shows impending loss of control of the disease. This is accomplished by RT-qPCR quantitation of *BCR-ABL1* transcript levels. One mechanism of resistance to treatment is selection for *BCR-ABL1* clones carrying mutations within the fusion gene which confer resistance to TKIs. A particular mutation, called T315I, is resistant to several TKIs. However, a third-generation TKI, ponatinib, has been specifically developed to overcome this.

Some patients in blast crisis may need to be treated with conventional chemotherapy and a TKI to achieve a second chronic phase. In most patients, the blast crisis resembles AML but in about a fifth of patients, the blasts are lymphoid. For the minority of patients presenting with blast crisis or who are resistant to multiple TKIs, transplant remains an important treatment modality, and a number of allogeneic stem cell transplants are still performed for this indication.

Polycythaemia vera

The second myeloproliferative neoplasm to discuss is polycythaemia vera (PV), a chronic clonal disorder causing excessive proliferation of the erythroid series, often accompanied by an increase in granulocyte and platelet counts. The underlying pathophysiology relates to the finding of an activating mutation in the *JAK2* gene, a key component of the JAK-STAT

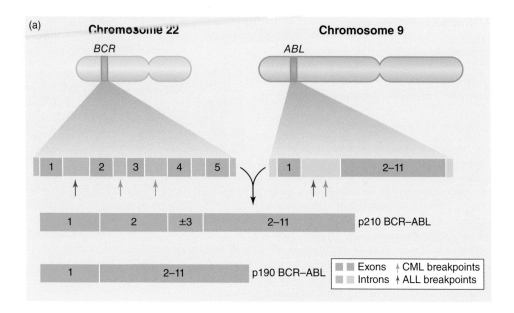

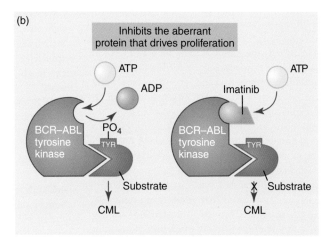

Figure 8.7 (a) Chromosomal breakpoints responsible for the *BCR-ABL* fusion gene. (b) Diagram showing the mechanism of action of imatinib. This drug inhibits the phosphorylation by *BCR-ABL* of tyrosine in protein (shown in green) and thereby interferes with its leukaemogenic effects.

signalling pathway which translates the effect of erythropoietin binding to the epo receptor on erythroid precursor membranes. This results in autonomous proliferation of the erythroid series, and the primary clinical manifestation is a markedly elevated haemoglobin and haematocrit.

Clinical features

Polycythaemia vera has an insidious onset, usually presenting late in life (rarely before 40 years). The main presenting symptoms relate to the considerable rise in red cell count and resulting increase in blood viscosity and include headache, dizziness and sometimes stroke. Pruritus, particularly after a hot bath, is a characteristic symptom. There is a marked tendency for patients to develop thrombosis, although there may also paradoxically be an increased likelihood of bleeding due to platelet dysfunction. Thromboses may occur at unusual sites, including within the mesenteric, portal or splenic veins. The principal signs are plethora (florid, dusky red colour of the face), splenomegaly and hepatomegaly. Erythromelalgia (increased skin temperature, burning sensation and redness) may occur in the extremities.

Laboratory findings and natural history

The red cell count and haemoglobin concentration are increased; haemoglobin values of 180–240 g/L are common and the packed cell volume (PCV) or haematocrit, by definition, is over 0.48 in females and 0.52 in males. An increase in the granulocyte count occurs in many patients and about 50% have an elevated platelet count. Polymerase chain reaction for the *JAK2* V617F mutation is central to investigation and is seen in at least 95% of patients. About 1–2% of cases have a mutation within exon 12 of the *JAK2* gene and a tiny proportion of patients meet the clinical criteria for PV but have no identifiable mutation. In all these cases, a suppressed erythropoietin level is normally seen.

Most patients with polycythaemia vera will remain well, provided that the haematocrit is controlled to <0.45 by venesection.

Differential diagnosis

Secondary erythrocytosis is the main differential diagnosis for polycythaemia vera. In secondary erythrocytosis, the prompt to red cell production is outside the marrow, and investigation will usually reveal an elevated (rather than suppressed) erythropoietin level. Long-standing hypoxia caused by cardiopulmonary disease or living at high altitudes will lead to an increased red cell mass and therefore a high haemoglobin and haematocrit by this mechanism (see Chapter 3). Rarely, epo may also be autonomously secreted by some renal tumours or in polycystic kidney disease. However, the elevated haematocrit and haemoglobin are usually the only haematological abnormality; where neutrophilia, thrombocytosis and splenomegaly are also found, polycythaemia vera is more likely.

Some patients may have a high haematocrit as a result of a reduction in the plasma volume. This is associated with diuretic therapy, heavy smoking, obesity and alcohol consumption. Patients with this so-called *relative* or *apparent erythrocytosis* will be negative for the *JAK2* V617F mutation and will typically have a normal epo level. Where uncertainty exists about the cause of polycythaemia following investigation including *JAK2* mutation analysis and epo levels, the red cell mass can be formally measured using isotope dilution methods, and bone marrow histology may be helpful.

Treatment

Options for treatment in polycythaemia vera include simple venesection, aiming to lower the haematocrit to below 0.45, thus reducing the risk of thrombotic episodes. In the early stages, this may have to be performed at least twice weekly. Low-dose aspirin is also used to minimize the risk of thrombosis. Patients with significant neutrophilia or thrombocytosis can be treated with cytoreductive therapy using oral chemotherapy agents such as hydroxycarbamide or interferon α, which can also selectively suppress the malignant myeloid clone. The JAK1/2 inhibitor ruxolitinib is used for those patients responding inadequately or intolerant of hydroxycarbamide.

Prognosis

The prognosis is normally good for patients with PV, and many patients may live for decades. In about 30% of patients, the marrow may become increasingly fibrotic (secondary myelofibrosis), leading to a fall in the haematocrit, increasing splenomegaly and often a requirement for blood transfusion in the later stages. About 5% of patients may develop AML.

Essential thrombocythaemia (ET)

This is a clonal myeloproliferative neoplasm that chiefly involves the megakaryocyte lineage. The disorder is classically associated with a marked rise in the platelet count, with the haemoglobin concentration and the neutrophil count typically being unaffected. Many patients are diagnosed by the incidental finding of thrombocytosis during the course of a routine blood count. The difficulty arises in differentiating this condition from the more common reactive causes of thrombocytosis (Box 8.3) and specific diagnostic criteria exist to help with this (see Box 8.4).

Genetic tests for clonal disorders are very useful in confirming the diagnosis of ET. Approximately 50% of patients with ET have the common *JAK2* mutation that has been identified in patients with polycythaemia vera (and also in primary myelofibrosis, see below); it remains unclear how this single mutation can give rise to these three distinct disease entities, though the allele burden of mutant *JAK2* is thought to be important. In those cases that are *JAK2* mutation negative, some will have a mutation in the calreticulin gene, *CALR*. A smaller number will have a mutation in the thrombopoietin receptor gene, *MPL*.

Box 8.3 Causes of thrombocytosis

Reactive:
- Haemorrhage, haemolysis, trauma, surgery, postpartum, recovery from thrombocytopenia
- Acute and chronic infections
- Chronic inflammatory disease (e.g. ulcerative colitis, rheumatoid arthritis)
- Malignant disease (e.g. carcinoma, Hodgkin lymphoma, some forms of myelodysplasia)
- Splenectomy and splenic atrophy
- Iron deficiency anaemia

Chronic myeloproliferative disorders:
- Essential thrombocythaemia
- Polycythaemia vera
- Chronic myeloid leukaemia
- Myelofibrosis

Box 8.4 Diagnostic criteria for essential thrombocythaemia

- Platelet count over 450×10^9/L (sustained).
- Essential thrombocythaemia bone marrow changes – proliferation of megakaryocytes with typical morphological features.
- Does not meet criteria for diagnosis of polycythaemia vera, myelofibrosis, chronic myeloid leukaemia or myelodysplastic syndromes.
- Presence of *JAK2* (50–60%), *MPL* (5%) or calreticulin *(CALR)* (25–30%) mutation.
- In the absence of a clonal marker, no reactive cause for thrombocytosis, normal iron stores and typical bone marrow features.

Clinical features

This is a disorder that affects older patients, usually presenting with thrombotic or bleeding complications. Many patients are asymptomatic at presentation. Older patients seem to be at greater risk of thrombosis, particularly arterial. The main thrombotic complications are as follows.

- Erythromelalgia and digital ischaemia: erythromelalgia is characterized by intense burning and pain in the extremities. The pain is increased by exercise, warmth or dependency. The extremities are warm with mottled erythema. Digital ischaemia mainly affects the toes. Such vascular

insufficiency sometimes leads to gangrene and loss of function.
- Stroke.
- Hepatic and portal vein thrombosis: the myeloproliferative disorders are the most common causes of hepatic vein thrombosis (Budd–Chiari syndrome).

In addition to thrombotic complications, paradoxically patients with ET, particularly those with a dramatically raised platelet count (over 1500×10^9/L), are at considerably increased risk of bleeding.

Laboratory findings

A raised platelet count, sometimes over 1000×10^9/L, is characteristic of the disorder. The bone marrow shows increased cellularity and plentiful megakaryocytes, often with atypical morphology. Certain criteria must be satisfied before the diagnosis can be entertained and these are listed in Box 8.4.

Treatment

There may not be any necessity to treat a young asymptomatic patient and most physicians suggest a risk-based approach. Patients over the age of 60 years with a markedly raised platelet count or with a history of thrombosis should be considered for active treatment. The following agents have been used.

- Simple oral chemotherapy with hydroxycarbamide – this is the most common treatment used.
- α-Interferon, which reduces platelet counts but may cause unacceptable side-effects such as fatigue, fever, pyrexia and depression. It is the treatment of choice in women of child-bearing age because of its relative safety in pregnancy, and may be useful in younger patients.
- Anagrelide, an agent that inhibits megakaryocyte maturation and does not affect the white cell count; its cardiac side-effect profile means it is less frequently used.

Antiplatelet drugs such as aspirin can be highly effective in patients at risk of thrombotic episodes. They may be associated with haemorrhage and should not be used in patients with a bleeding tendency.

JAK inhibitors such as ruxolitinib are being assessed but are not yet in routine clinical use.

Prognosis

The disease tends to be stable for decades, and life expectancy is similar to the normal population.

There is a risk of transformation to secondary myelofibrosis, however (about 5% at 10 years), and also to AML (1–4%).

Primary myelofibrosis

This clonal myeloproliferative neoplasm is characterized by the development of extensive bone marrow reticulin fibrosis. This fibrosis is itself reactive and is thought to be secondary to the clonal abnormal haematopoiesis, particularly of the megakaryocytic lineage. At the molecular level, approximately 50% of patients with primary myelofibrosis harbour the same *JAK2* mutation that has been identified in patients with primary polycythaemia. A further quarter of affected patients are found to have mutations in the calreticulin gene, *CALR* (and these patients tend to be younger with less aggressive disease). In a smaller number of patients, mutations affecting the thrombopoietin receptor gene (*MPL*) have been described. Interestingly, the mutations and their frequency are very similar to those found in essential thrombocythaemia.

The disorder may transform to AML in about 25% of cases. Although the principal site of extramedullary haematopoiesis is the spleen or liver, other sites such as the lymph nodes, adrenal or dura may be involved. Secondary myelofibrosis may also arise on a background of PV or ET.

Clinical features

This disorder usually presents in patients over the age of 50 years, but can occasionally occur in younger patients. Patients present with constitutional symptoms such as weight loss, night sweats or fever. Massive splenomegaly may be seen as a result of extramedullary haematopoiesis, and other presenting features may include splenic pain or early satiety. Symptoms resulting from bone marrow failure as the marrow becomes fibrotic will include fatigue, shortness of breath and palpitations as a consequence of anaemia. Occasional patients present with gout as a consequence of hyperuricaemia resulting from the high cell turnover.

Laboratory findings

Normochromic normocytic anaemia is found in most patients with myelofibrosis. Leucocytosis and thrombocytosis are common findings, although the total white cell count is not usually as high as that found in CML and is rarely over 40×10^9/L. Inspection of the blood film is often diagnostic. The blood film typically shows the presence of normoblasts and myelocytes (i.e. a leucoerythroblastic picture, with the presence of teardrop poikilocytes; Figure 8.8). Bone marrow aspiration is usually unsuccessful because of the fibrosis, resulting in a dry tap. The bone marrow biopsy shows myeloproliferation with granulocytic and megakaryocytic hyperplasia together with fibrosis, which may be dense (Figure 8.9). Genetic analysis for *JAK2*, *CALR* and *MPL* mutations is essential, and may also provide prognostic information (patients with *CALR* mutated tend to have a more favourable prognosis). Screening for other mutated genes, including *TP53*, may also offer important prognostic information and is routinely performed.

Treatment

How myelofibrosis is treated depends upon the prognosis. Those with lower risk disease or unfit patients may be managed with supportive care including blood transfusions, erythropoietin and hydroxycarbamide (which may be useful in patients with a significant leucocytosis). Other agents used include danazol (which may improve anaemia), immunomodulatory agents such as lenalidomide, and prednisolone. Splenectomy may be considered for patients with severe symptomatic splenomegaly and occasionally radiotherapy may be used in patients unfit for surgery, although the overall benefit is usually modest.

Ruxolitinib, the JAK inhibitor, has been shown to reduce spleen size, improve constitutional symptoms and quality of life, and increase survival. It is generally used in higher risk patients as first-line treatment.

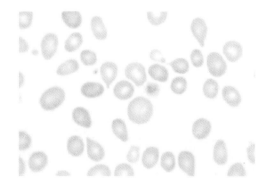

Figure 8.8 Blood film of a patient with idiopathic myelofibrosis showing several teardrop-shaped poikilocytes and an abnormally large platelet. MGG stain.

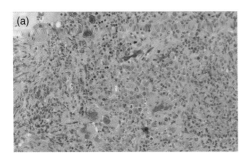
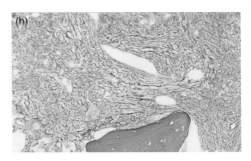

Figure 8.9 (a) Trephine biopsy of the bone marrow of a patient with myelofibrosis The marrow is hypercellular, with evidence of cellular streaming and atypical megakaryocytes. Haematoxylin and eosin stain, ×20 magnification. (b) Section of the same trephine biopsy showing increased fibrosis (reticulin).

Patients do not have to have the *JAK2* mutation to benefit. It may lead to transient worsening of cytopenias, but is normally well tolerated. Overall, the increase in survival is modest; it does not lead to prolonged remissions, and should not be confused in this respect with imatinib in CML.

The only curative option is allogeneic stem cell transplant, and this can cure around 40–50% of patients with myelofibrosis. Patients at high risk of transformation to AML or a poor prognosis who are young enough (under 70) and fit should be considered for this. Post transplant, patients often have poor engraftment with cytopenias which may last for several months, and the risk of primary graft failure is higher than in other conditions.

Prognosis

Prognosis depends upon the patient's age, presence of constitutional symptoms, degree of cytopenias, karyotype and molecular mutations. Standardised scoring systems exist which help estimate the prognosis for an individual patient. The average prognosis is around 5 years, although some patients may only live a few months, and some patients may live 10–20 years.

9

Neoplastic disorders of lymphoid cells

LEARNING OBJECTIVES

After reading this chapter, you should be able to:

✔ understand the pathological changes, clinical presentation, investigation and principles of management of Hodgkin lymphoma

✔ understand the pathological changes, clinical manifestations and the basic principles of treatment of acute lymphoblastic leukaemia

✔ understand the pathological changes, clinical manifestations and basic principles of treatment of the more common non-Hodgkin lymphomas, chronic lymphocytic leukaemia (CLL), diffuse large B-cell lymphoma (DLBCL) and follicular lymphoma.

Lymphomas are the fifth most common malignancy in the UK and one of the more common malignancies affecting younger people. They are frequently treatable, and in some cases curable, and can present with clinical symptoms and signs in any organ system. As well as being of major clinical significance, they are also biologically fascinating, and major steps forward have been taken in the last few years toward a better understanding of their pathogenesis and management.

Although the chapter which follows is divided into sections focused on Hodgkin and non-Hodgkin lymphoma, many elements are common to both subtypes. Concepts of staging and supportive care, relevant to all lymphoma types, are discussed in Chapter 6.

Hodgkin lymphoma

Hodgkin lymphoma is one of the more common lymphomas affecting young people, and in many cases is potentially curable. As well as its clear clinical signifi-cance, its underlying biology is also of interest. Hodgkin lymphoma is unusual in that the bulk of the tumour mass comprises a polyclonal inflammatory infiltrate and variable fibrosis, with the malignant cells, the Reed–Sternberg or Hodgkin cells (Figure 9.1) being relatively sparse. Indeed, from its first descrip-tion (accredited to Dr Thomas Hodgkin of Guy's Hospital in 1832 after the study of affected lymph glands in postmortem cases), this disorder was termed Hodgkin *disease* as its underlying cell of origin was unclear; it was only in the 1990s that microdissection of the Reed–Sternberg cells allowed them to be for-mally identified as abnormal B cells, with rearrangedimmunoglobin V genes. The term Hodgkin *disease* is now correctly replaced by Hodgkin *lymphoma*.

Under the term Hodgkin lymphoma are recognized two clinically and biologically different entities: clas-sic Hodgkin lymphoma, and non-classic Hodgkin lymphoma, also known as nodular lymphocyte-predominant Hodgkin lymphoma (NLPHL), which has a chronic relapsing course and often behaves more like a low grade non-Hodgkin lymphoma.

Haematology Lecture Notes, Eleventh Edition. Deborah Hay, Andrew King and Michael Desborough.
© 2023 John Wiley & Sons Ltd. Published 2023 by John Wiley & Sons Ltd.
Companion website: www.wiley.com/go/Hay/Haematology/11e

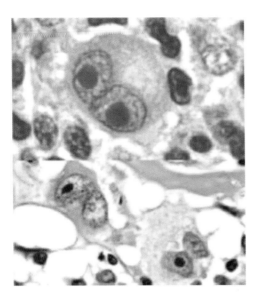

Figure 9.1 Photomicrograph showing Reed–Sternberg cells from a case of Hodgkin lymphoma.

Incidence and aetiology

Whereas the incidence of non-Hodgkin lymphoma increased in the 1980s and 1990s, the incidence of Hodgkin lymphoma has remained stable at about 3 per 100 000 population. It is more common in men than in women (2:1 predominance) and increases in incidence with age, peaking in the third decade, followed by a decline. There appears to be a second peak in later life which characteristically has a worse prognosis.

The aetiology of Hodgkin lymphoma is unknown. The apparent geographical clustering of cases that has been reported has suggested an infectious aetiol-ogy and many efforts have been made to identify likely culprits. Epstein–Barr virus (EBV) has long remained a favoured possible cause, because similar age groups are affected by both Hodgkin lymphoma and glandular fever. There is some evidence that EBV may have a part to play in the aetiology of Hodgkin lymphoma, supported by the finding of clonal EBV DNA in 30–40% of cases.

Clinical features

Lymph node enlargement is the most common presentation, usually affecting the neck and mediastinum (Figure 9.2). The cervical nodes are affected in 60–70% of cases, axillary nodes in 10–15% of cases, and inguinal nodes in 6–12% of cases. Splenomegaly and hepatomegaly may be seen. Mediastinal involvement is found in up to 10% of patients and may be associated with pleural effusions or superior vena cava obstruction; patients may present with cough, chest pain or shortness of breath. Spread is mainly along the lymph vessels; hence lymph node involvement tends to be contiguous. Sweats, fever, weight loss and pruritus may occur although their absence should never be used to exclude lymphoma. Alcohol-induced pain in affected lymph nodes is pathognomonic, but rare.

The staging system using cross-sectional imaging is shown in Chapter 6, and is also used for non-Hodgkin lymphoma. A positron emission tomography/computed tomography (PET-CT) is always obtained where possible in order to stage patients accurately, and for monitoring response to treatment. A full blood count, erythrocyte sedimentation rate (ESR), liver function tests, renal and bone profile and lactate dehydrogenase (LDH) are all necessary and may confer prognostic information.

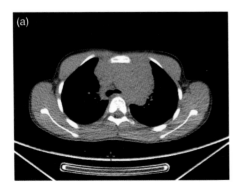
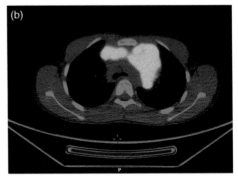

Figure 9.2 A mediastinal mass visible on CT imaging in a patient with Hodgkin lymphoma (a). This is FDG avid (b).

Treatment

Classic Hodgkin lymphoma

The majority (>80%) of patients with classic Hodgkin lymphoma are cured with front-line treatment, the overall survival rate typically being >90–95%. The goal of treatment for Hodgkin lymphoma is therefore cure, while minimizing complications.

Early-stage disease (stages IA–IIA) can be effectively treated with abbreviated chemotherapy, often together with localized radiotherapy. Advanced disease (stages IIB–IV) is usually treated with full combination chemotherapy; radiotherapy is reserved to treat residual masses or given after completion of chemotherapy to areas previously involved by bulky disease. Modern treatment is based on the need to attain a high cure rate, minimize the toxicity of treatment and preserve fertility. The high 'cure' rate in Hodgkin lymphoma may be at the cost of a higher death rate from second malignancies and other toxicities and the use of alkylating agents and radiotherapy is likely to contribute to this excess risk. This increase in death rate from causes other than Hodgkin lymphoma is graphically illustrated in Figure 9.3. After 15 years from diagnosis, mortality from causes other than Hodgkin lymphoma is greater than deaths from the lymphoma itself, although this trend may change as patients are treated with modern chemotherapy regimens that aim to reduce long-term toxicity. Irradiation of peripubertal breast tissue is thought to put patients at particularly high risk of breast cancer.

Regimens containing doxorubicin (also called adriamycin), e.g. ABVD (doxorubicin, bleomycin, vinblastine, dacarbazine), are favoured for initial treatment because of the low incidence of secondary leukaemia and the fact that most patients, both male and female, remain fertile. ABVD is myelosuppressive and two drugs of this four-drug regimen are associated with potentially serious side-effects: the use of

bleomycin can cause significant pulmonary toxicity and exposure to high doses of anthracyclines is known to cause cardiomyopathy. Older patients are at higher risk of bleomycin-induced lung toxicity and bleomycin is normally limited or omitted in those aged >60. The latter two problems can be avoided by close monitoring and discontinuation of the drug at the first sign of complications. Some centres prefer more intensive treatment upfront incorporating more chemotherapy drugs. These have a higher cure rate but may lead to more short- and longer-term toxicity.

All patients with Hodgkin lymphoma should be staged before treatment with whole-body PET-CT. In advanced stage disease, repeat imaging after the first two cycles of chemotherapy is routine to assess response and is now standard of care. Patients not in remission after two cycles of chemotherapy have been found to have a poor outcome and may be switched to more intensive chemotherapy regimens. Those in a metabolic remission and receiving ABVD may have the bleomycin omitted from future cycles. This 'risk-adapted' programme of management means that patients may avoid unnecessarily toxic treatments.

For the 20% who fail to respond to initial therapy, or who relapse, further chemotherapy containing a platinum agent followed by high-dose therapy with peripheral blood stem cell rescue may be curative. Approximately 50% of such patients respond well to this approach.

Brentuximab vedotin is an anti-CD30 antibody conjugated to a microtubule-disrupting agent and may be effective in patients resistant to conventional chemotherapy. It is normally well tolerated aside from peripheral neuropathy. Brentuximab is also very effective in frontline treatment when combined with AVD.

A newer approach to treatment has emerged from studies of immune checkpoint activity in Hodgkin lymphoma. This tumour often expresses high levels of the 'programmed death-1' ligand (PD-L1) which regulates the immune response and allows tumours to

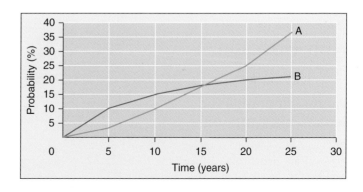

Figure 9.3 Actuarial risk of death from Hodgkin lymphoma (b) or other causes (a) in patients treated for Hodgkin lymphoma.

evade the T-cell immune response, PD-1 1 blockade is thus highly effective in the management of relapsed Hodgkin lymphoma and offers an option for patients who are refractory to multiple lines of chemotherapy. Drugs used include nivolumab and pembrolizumab.

For the minority of patients refractory to multiple lines of therapy, allogeneic stem cell transplant may be curative.

Prognosis

A number of attempts have been made to predict outcome in patients treated for Hodgkin lymphoma. The prognosis is worse for males, older patients, patients with advanced disease and those with a low serum albumin concentration, anaemia and leucocytosis. Understanding prognostic factors enables more intensive treatment to be given to patients with a predicted worse outcome, while those with a good prognosis may be spared unnecessary toxicity and adverse late effects.

Nodular lymphocyte-predominant Hodgkin lymphoma

Nodular lymphocyte-predominant Hodgkin lymphoma is a rare subtype, accounting for approximately 5% of all cases of Hodgkin lymphoma. It is most common in middle-aged males. The pathological and clinical features differ from classic Hodgkin lymphoma. The disease-defining lymphocyte-predominant Hodgkin cells express CD20, and do not express CD30, unlike the Reed–Sternberg cell, and the clinical course of the disease tends to be rather indolent, similar to low-grade NHL. There is a risk of late relapses and histological transformation into more aggressive forms of NHL. Overall, however, the prognosis is excellent, with the majority of patients experiencing long remissions after minimal treatment, which may include involved field radiotherapy and combination chemotherapy for more advanced stage disease.

Non-Hodgkin lymphomas

Acute lymphoblastic leukaemia/lymphoma

Precursor lymphoblastic neoplasms of B- or T-cell type typically present as a leukaemia with circulating blast cells (acute lymphoblastic leukaemia, ALL)

and symptoms of marrow failure. By definition, patients have >20% blasts in the bone marrow, but the marrow is often heavily infiltrated with blasts, which are also present in the peripheral blood (Figure 9.4). Sometimes, patients may have disease confined to the lymph nodes with limited or absent bone marrow disease – this is termed lymphoblastic lymphoma.

The disorder results from clonal proliferation of cells from the earliest stages of lymphoid maturation (i.e. B or T blast cells). B-cell leukaemia blast cells have a phenotype defined by the presence of CD19, CD79a, CD10, CD34 and terminal deoxynucleotidyl transferase (TdT). T-cell leukaemia is TdT positive and also expresses T cell markers (CD1a, CD2-8).

Cytogenetic analysis provides important prognostic information. Treatment regimens are based on risk stratification and therefore cytogenetics is an important part of the investigations at presentation. Hyperdiploidy (increased numbers of chromosomes beyond the diploid state) and t(12;21) generally carry a good prognosis, whereas the Philadelphia

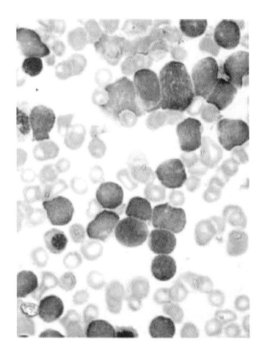

Figure 9.4 Bone marrow smear from a patient with acute lymphoblastic leukaemia. The blasts are small or medium sized and have scanty cytoplasm. The nuclei have fine but densely packed, homogeneous-appearing chromatin and the nucleoli are small.

chromosome t(9;22), hypodiploidy and rearrangements of the *MLL* gene carry a poor prognosis. As well as cytogenetics, mutations in some genes also provide prognostic information, including *TP53*.

Clinical and laboratory features

Acute lymphoblastic leukaemia is the most common childhood cancer, but can present at any age. In children, the peak incidence is between the ages of 2 and 4 years. The clinical manifestations and laboratory findings are listed in Box 9.1; most of the clinical manifestations can be explained in terms of bone marrow failure secondary to bone marrow infiltration. A small proportion of patients may have CNS disease at diagnosis, presenting with headache, altered GCS or seizures. Aside from genetic features, adverse prognostic features include a high white cell count at diagnosis (>50) or age >10 or <1.

Treatment

Treatment of childhood acute leukaemia has improved greatly, largely thanks to the results of clinical trials that have conducted over the last 30–40 years. Risk stratification based on prognostic factors, including diagnostic features and dynamic measurable residual disease (see below), is used to determine the protocols with which children and adults with ALL are treated, though the general schema is outlined here. Teenagers and young adults (typically up to age 30) are managed using the more intensive paediatric protocols.

1 *Induction*. The aim of induction chemotherapy is to clear the bone marrow of leukaemia blast cells to give a morphologically normal bone marrow and normal blood counts.
2 *Consolidation*. Consolidation therapy reduces the leukaemia cell burden further and uses a combination of moderately intensive treatment after normal haematopoiesis has been restored with induction chemotherapy.
3 *CNS prophylaxis*. Without appropriate CNS-directed treatment, patients with ALL will relapse in the CNS. A phase of prophylactic treatment to prevent CNS involvement is always given. This can be achieved by administration of high-dose chemotherapy drugs such as methotrexate, which cross the blood–brain barrier, or by direct administration of methotrexate into the cerebrospinal fluid (intrathecal). On all protocols, several doses of intrathecal chemotherapy are given.
4 *Maintenance therapy*. The final treatment phase is maintenance therapy. Continuous oral and intermittent intravenous chemotherapy is given over 2–3 years with intrathecal chemotherapy every 3 months.

High-risk ALL may require intensification of chemotherapy and, particularly in adults, an allogeneic stem cell transplant. For patients who relapse or who are refractory to treatment, newer targeted agents can be used, including bispecific antibodies and antibody–drug conjugates. CAR T cell therapy (see Chapter 12) has also been used in these patients with good effect.

Box 9.1 Acute lymphoblastic leukaemia

Clinical features of ALL

Symptoms and their pathological basis:
- Weakness, tiredness, malaise, lassitude caused by anaemia
- Bruising and bleeding secondary to thrombocytopenia
- Otitis media, pharyngitis, pneumonia or fever from bacterial infection caused by neutropenia
- Bone pain or limping as a result of marrow infiltration
- Enlarged lymph nodes
- Shortness of breath due to a mediastinal mass
- Testicular swelling (a testicular examination should always be performed at diagnosis)
- Headache and vomiting resulting from CNS involvement leading to increased intracranial pressure

Physical findings:
- Pallor
- Petechial haemorrhages, purpura and bruising
- Lymphadenopathy
- Hepatosplenomegaly
- Bone tenderness
- Fever

Laboratory features of ALL
- Anaemia
- Neutropenia
- Thrombocytopenia
- Blood film may show circulating blast cells
- Bone marrow usually heavily infiltrated with blast cells (>20%)
- Recurring cytogenetic abnormalities (~80% cases)

Measurable residual disease

Response to treatment in ALL is assessed on bone marrow biopsies after cycles of chemotherapy. Even when the bone marrow appears morphologically normal and cytogenetic abnormalities are no longer detectable, small numbers of tumour cells may still be present. The amount of detectable residual leukaemia cells after treatment cycles is referred to as measurable (or minimal) residual disease (MRD) – see Chapter 8.

Randomized studies have shown the prognostic importance of MRD, and its measurement allows risk-adapted therapy. For example, patients with undetectable or very low MRD levels after induction may have chemotherapy de-escalated; patients with high levels of MRD despite chemotherapy may require treatment intensification or an allogeneic stem cell transplant.

Prognosis and long-term considerations

There is considerable variation in the prognosis dependent upon the genetic and clinical features at diagnosis and the age of the patient. Cure rates for children and young adults are very good, reaching 80–90%, normally with chemotherapy alone. Cure rates for adults are less good, with around 40% of patients surviving 5 years. The challenge for the future is to define risk groups more effectively with continued integration of MRD allowing ongoing individualization of therapy.

Given the excellent cure rates in children and young adults, long-term effects from treatment are increasingly recognized. Specific concerns are avascular necrosis of the bones due to high-dose steroids, the long-term risk associated with anthracycline use, and the potential risk of infertility and secondary cancers. Many centres now have late effects clinics to monitor and treat these complications.

Lymphoblastic lymphoma

This represents the lymphomatous equivalent of ALL (i.e. there is little peripheral blood or bone marrow involvement). It has very similar features to ALL but there are a number of characteristic clinical features: it is more common in adolescent males and patients frequently present with a mediastinal mass. Patients have <20% blasts in their bone marrow, otherwise they are classified as having ALL. Lymphoblastic lymphoma is treated using the same protocols as for ALL.

Diffuse large B-cell lymphoma

Diffuse large B-cell lymphoma (DLBCL) is the most common high-grade lymphoma. It typifies an aggressive but potentially curable lymphoma, and represents approximately one-third of all lymphomas. The disorder occurs at all ages but becomes more common in later life. Patients present with rapidly progressive disease, featuring night sweats, fever, weight loss and lymphadenopathy or with extranodal lymphoma involving sites such as the gastrointestinal tract, testis, brain or bone.

Histologically, the disorder is characterized by the presence of sheets of large cells of B-cell origin. The disorder probably includes a variety of different lymphoma types and in this sense is a catch-all category for those lymphomas that do not obviously fit into other definitions. At least two different types (activated B cell [ABC] type and germinal centre [GC]) of DLBCL are described. Translocations between the IgH locus on chromosome 14 and other genes (*BCL2*, *MYC* and *BCL6*) are sometimes present. DLBCL which has two translocations where there is overexpression of both BCL2 and MYC (so-called 'double-hit' lymphoma) has a particularly poor prognosis. The immunophenotype is CD20+, CD79+, CD5–, CD23–, CD10– and sIgM+. The immunophenotype may also reflect the cell of origin (e.g. GC or ABC type).

A variety of clinical and laboratory findings are relevant to the outcome of therapy and make up the International Prognostic Index (IPI), including age, performance status, stage, number of extranodal sites and serum LDH.

Treatment and prognosis

Treatment is with combination chemotherapy, which can induce remission in approximately 80% of cases, and as many as 70% of patients will attain a sustained remission beyond 3 years. The combination of cyclophosphamide, doxorubicin (hydroxydaunorubicin), vincristine (oncovin) and prednisolone (CHOP) with the anti-CD20 antibody rituximab has been the gold standard against which other treatments are judged, with the addition of rituximab showing a significant survival advantage over CHOP alone. For localized disease (stage I and stage II), 3–4 courses of R-CHOP are given, in some cases with radiotherapy. Advanced disease is treated with six cycles. Response to treatment is normally monitored with PET-CT during treatment and then following completion. Radiotherapy is often given to sites of bulky disease or residual masses after the completion of chemotherapy. Some centres prefer more intensive chemotherapy regimens for aggressive or very high-risk lymphomas.

Relapsed or refractory patients are treated with high-dose platinum-based chemotherapy, consolidated with an autologous stem cell transplant, and up to 40% will obtain durable remissions. In patients with relapsed or resistant disease, newer therapies include chimeric antigen receptor (CAR) T-cell therapy (e.g. with a CAR directed against CD19) or an antibody–drug conjugate directed against the B-cell marker CD79.

Burkitt lymphoma

Burkitt lymphoma is a high-grade lymphoma characterized by its very aggressive clinical course. The pathogenesis focuses on activation of the *MYC* oncogene, as described in Chapter 6. All cases have a translocation of the *MYC* gene on chromosome 8 to one of the immunoglobulin genes (for the heavy chain, κ light chain or λ light chain) on chromosome 14, 22 or 2 – t(8;14), t(2;8) and t(8;22). These translocations bring the *MYC* gene under the control of the relevant immunoglobulin gene enhancers, resulting in increased *MYC* transcription, such that every neoplastic cell is actively dividing.

Burkitt lymphoma presents in one of three main forms: endemic, sporadic or a type associated with immunodeficiency states. The endemic form mainly affects children in East Africa, presents with a jaw or facial bone tumour and is nearly always positive for Epstein–Barr virus. Infection with malaria is thought to play an important part in the pathogenesis of this form of Burkitt lymphoma, probably by chronic antigen stimulation. Sporadic Burkitt lymphoma occurs in the West, is only sometimes EBV-positive and tends to present with extranodal disease, most commonly

an abdominal mass though breast, gonads, CNS and bone marrow are other commonly affected sites. Burkitt lymphoma also occurs in HIV-positive patients.

The pathology is characteristic, with diffuse infiltration by small to medium B cells, a very high proliferation rate of ~100% as described above and a high rate of apoptosis, which leads to the characteristic 'starry sky' appearance: the presence of macrophages scavenging apoptotic material leaves 'holes' in the otherwise uniform sheet of proliferating B cells (Figure 9.5). The immunophenotype of Burkitt lymphoma is of germinal centre type, CD19+, CD20+, BCL2– and CD10+.

The treatment of Burkitt lymphoma is usually successful, with multi-agent chemotherapy giving a >90% cure rate for patients with limited stage disease; those with more advanced disease can also be cured using this approach. Tumour lysis syndrome is a risk – see Box 9.4. CNS prophylactic treatment is necessary in all cases.

Chronic lymphocytic leukaemia

Chronic lymphocytic leukaemia (CLL) is a low-grade neoplastic lymphoid disorder characterized by the accumulation of small mature lymphocytes in the blood (Figure 9.6), bone marrow and lymphoid tissues. This is the most common leukaemia seen in the Western world and tends to affect adults over the age of 50 years with a peak incidence between 60 and 80. The disorder is much less common in China, Japan and South-East Asia.

The cells that give rise to the disorder express the B-cell markers CD19 and CD20 but also aberrantly express the T-cell marker CD5, meaning that flow cytometry can often be useful in making this diagnosis. Clonality can be established by skewed κ/λ light chain expression. Cytogenetic and molecular

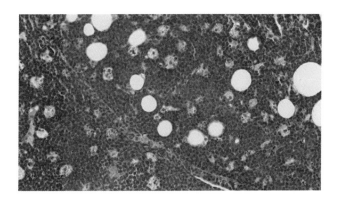

Figure 9.5 Histological section showing Burkitt lymphoma. As well as the well-demarcated fat spaces within the biopsy, the sheets of uniform medium-sized B cells are interspersed with macrophages and apoptotic cells – the classic 'starry sky' morphology.

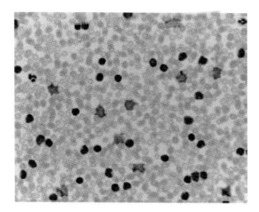

Figure 9.6 Blood film in a patient with chronic lymphocytic leukaemia. Note the presence of increased numbers of small lymphocytes and some smear cells.

studies provide prognostic information, with the most important findings being deletion of 17p (which contains the *TP53* gene) or a *TP53* mutation. The clinical and laboratory features of CLL are summarized in Box 9.2.

Autoimmune phenomena may occur in patients with CLL. The most common manifestations are autoimmune haemolytic anaemia (AIHA) and immune thrombocytopenic purpura (ITP). Patients may rarely develop pure red cell aplasia or neutropenia. Acquired angio-oedema may also result from autoimmune antibodies against the C1 esterase inhibitor. The antibodies are not thought to be produced by the malignant B cells, but rather by dysregulation of bystander populations of normal B cells.

Chronic lymphocytic leukaemia has a predictable natural history. Most patients have only a lymphocytosis at the beginning of their illness and progress to develop lymphadenopathy, hepatosplenomegaly and finally bone marrow failure. It is the presence or absence of these features that determines the prognosis. In about 3% of CLL cases, transformation to DLBCL or, much more rarely, other forms of lymphoma may occur. This is called a Richter transformation and it carries an extremely poor prognosis.

Clonal B cells with the same atypical phenotype as CLL are found at low levels in the blood of many older people. This is called monoclonal B-cell lymphocytosis; all patients with CLL progress from this stage. For CLL to be diagnosed, the monoclonal B cell count has to be >5 × 10⁹/L.

Box 9.2 Chronic lymphocytic leukaemia

Clinical features of CLL
- Most patients are over 60 years of age
- Many patients are asymptomatic at diagnosis, presenting with a lymphocytosis on blood counts done for other reasons
- Patients may present with symptoms attributable to anaemia – tiredness and fatigue
- Bruising and bleeding secondary to thrombocytopenia
- Sinusitis, bacterial pneumonia, secondary to hypogammaglobulinaemia
- Night sweats, fever and weight loss are uncommon but may occur

Physical findings:
- Lymphadenopathy
- Hepatosplenomegaly

Laboratory features of CLL
- Monoclonal lymphocytosis is greater than 5×10^9/L
- In the more advanced stages of the disease there may be anaemia and thrombocytopenia
- The direct antiglobulin (Coombs) test may be positive
- Bone marrow aspirate and trephine biopsy demonstrate the extent of bone marrow infiltration; this is typically high
- Hypogammaglobulinaemia is a common finding – a small proportion of patients will have a monoclonal band on immunoelectrophoresis
- Immunophenotyping of the malignant lymphocytes shows expression of CD5, CD19, CD20, CD23 and CD79a and surface IgM (weakly positive); CD10 is negative

Hypogammaglobulinaemia

Patients with CLL commonly have an associated hypogammaglobulinaemia. Reductions in the serum levels of IgM, IgG and IgA may all occur and these predispose to infections, particularly of the respiratory tract, by capsulated organisms such as *Streptococcus pneumoniae* and *Haemophilus influenzae*. Replacement therapy with intravenous pooled human immunoglobulin and/or prophylactic antibiotics can reduce the frequency of respiratory tract infections in such patients.

Treatment

Since CLL is currently incurable with conventional therapies, patients with CLL who are asymptomatic do not require treatment; simple monitoring is sufficient. Indications for treatment include systemic symptoms such as sweats, fever, weight loss, cytopenias such as anaemia or significant lymphadenopathy. Many elderly patients may never require treatment.

For many years, chemotherapy agents including the anti-CD20 monoclonal antibody rituximab (widely used in many B-cell lymphomas), combined with cytotoxic chemotherapy such as fludarabine, cyclophosphamide, bendamustine or chlorambucil, were the mainstay of treatment. Modern treatment, however, consists of more targeted treatments which are used frontline. These include:

- Drugs which suppress signalling through the B-cell receptor (BCR). Inhibitors of the Bruton tyrosine kinase (BTK) including drugs such as ibrutinib and acalabrutinib lead to B-cell apoptosis and are highly effective, either in combination with monoclonal antibodies or as single agents, even in patients with

17p deletion or a *TP53* mutation. Side-effects include cytopenias, an increased risk of bleeding and cardiac arrhythmias, particularly atrial fibrillation.
- Inactivators of the PI3KD protein. Phosphoinositide 3-kinase (PI3K) is another critical enzyme in BCR signalling. Idelalisib blocks its activity and is consequently used in CLL. It is normally well tolerated.
- Drugs which suppress activity of BCL-2. This is expressed at a high level in most CLL cells and has anti-apoptotic effects. Venetoclax is a potent BCL-2 inhibitor and is used in combination with monoclonal antibodies with excellent efficacy and tolerability.
- New more effective anti-CD20 monoclonal antibodies include ofatumumab and obinutuzumab.

The B-cell receptor signalling is shown in Figure 9.7. BTK inhibitors are also used in other clonal B-cell

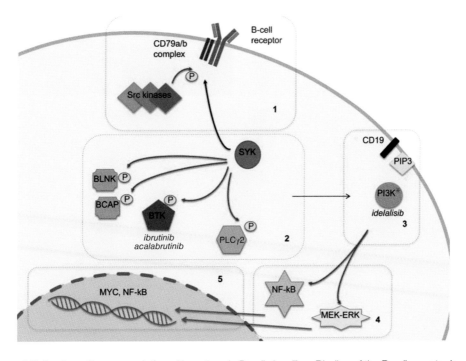

Figure 9.7 A schematic representation of key steps in B-cell signalling. Binding of the B-cell receptor by antigen induces a conformational change which exposes the immunoreceptor tyrosine-based activation motifs (ITAMs) on the associated CD79a/b complex. This means that these can be phosphorylated by the Src family kinases, Lyn, Fyn and Blk (Panel 1). This in turn creates a site to which the tyrosine kinase SYK can bind, with its resultant activation. SYK then goes on to phosphorylate phospholipase Cγ2 (PLCγ2) and Bruton tyrosine kinase (BTK), as well as B-cell linker (BLNK) and B-cell adaptor for phosphoinositide 3-kinase (BCAP) (Panel 2). These agents contribute to activation of the phosphoinositide-3 kinase (PI3K) (Panel 3). The PI3K pathway and BTK, along with additional signalling cascades, cause NK-κB activation, and activation of the MEK-ERK signalling cascades (Panel 4). The downstream effect is modulation of gene expression by transcription factors including NF-κB itself and MYC. Key stages in this process may be inhibited therapeutically (signified by the red asterisks). The BTK inhibitors ibrutinib and acalabrutinib and PI3K inhibitor idelalisib are in current clinical use.

disorders, including mantle cell lymphoma and lymphoplasmacytic lymphoma.

Allogeneic stem cell transplant is occasionally still used for patients with disease resistant to multiple agents although this is uncommon.

Prognosis

Many patients with early-stage CLL may never require treatment. For those who do, a typical pattern is response to treatment, typically for years, before a gradual relapse. The 5-year survival for all patients is >80%, and it is likely this will continue to improve with the newer targeted treatments. Richter transformation remains challenging to treat, with a prognosis normally measurable in months; a minority of patients may respond to therapy directed against DLBCL (R-CHOP) and then an allogeneic stem cell transplant.

Follicular lymphoma

Follicular lymphoma (FL) is another low-grade NHL which is relatively easy for the pathologist to identify because of its follicular growth pattern (Figure 9.8).

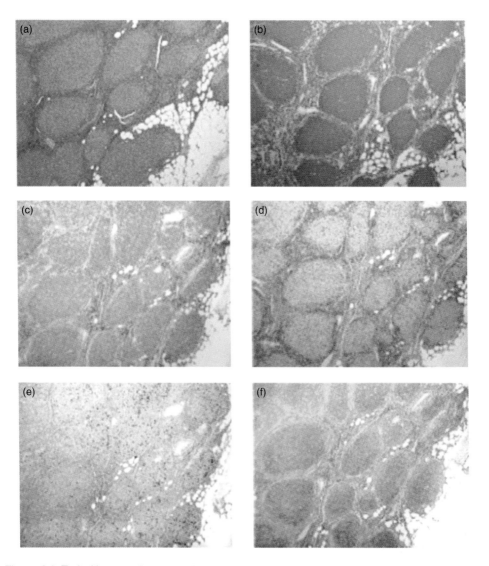

Figure 9.8 Typical immunophenotype of follicular lymphoma (paraffin section): (a) haematoxylin and eosin (H&E), (b) CD20, (c) bcl-2, (d) CD3, (e) Ki67 and (f) CD10.
Source: Courtesy of Professor Kevin Gatter.

As with the other low-grade lymphoproliferative diseases, this disorder is indolent in its clinical course but remains incurable. FL is associated with a translocation between chromosome 14 and 18, t(14;18), which leads to the upregulation of the antiapoptotic protein BCL-2. The t(14;18) translocation is thought to arise in early B cells, which then move into the germinal centre of the lymph node follicle where they acquire additional mutations, causing FL. The presence of the t(14;18) translocation is insufficient to cause FL on its own. In a proportion of cases, further additional mutations may cause the lymphoma to transform to a DLBCL type: this is high-grade transformation.

Follicular lymphoma is one of the most common types of lymphoma and accounts for 25% of all NHL. Most patients present with widespread painless lymphadenopathy, bone marrow infiltration and hepatosplenomegaly. Sometimes circulating FL cells may be seen in the peripheral blood. Occasionally, this lymphoma presents in an extranodal fashion, the gastrointestinal tract and the skin being among the sites where this may occur. The majority of patients will have stage III or IV disease at diagnosis. B symptoms may also occur. The immunophenotype is CD19+, CD20+, CD10+, BCL2+ and BCL6+.

The clinical course alternates between stable periods, when patients remain well, and periods of progressive disease requiring therapy. High-grade transformation occurs in 30% of patients and confers a poor prognosis. Rapidly enlarging lymph nodes are suggestive of this clinically.

Treatment and prognosis

For the 10% of patients with disease localized to one nodal area (or two nodal areas providing this can be encompassed in a single radiotherapy field), radiotherapy may be curative, with at least 60–70% of patients having no evidence of disease 10 years later. Patients require careful staging with both a bone marrow biopsy and PET-CT to ensure the disease is truly localized.

There is no evidence that early or intensive treatment of FL at presentation in advanced stage disease improves outcome. Therapy is required, however, in patients with systemic symptoms, organ failure or bulky disease. Typical first-line regimens include R-CVP (rituximab, cyclophosphamide, vincristine, prednisolone) and R-bendamustine. Anti-CD20 monoclonal antibodies may also be used as maintenance treatment to prolong remissions. Alternative combination chemotherapy agents can be used at relapse, and high-dose therapy with stem cell rescue or allografting (see Chapter 12) may be appropriate in selected patients. Future potential therapies include CAR T-cells directed against CD19, and bispecific antibodies, which bind both CD3 and CD20 and engage T cells with B cells including lymphoma cells.

The prognosis of FL is variable, ranging from 2 to 20 years. The median survival is about 10–12 years from diagnosis.

Lymphoplasmacytic lymphoma/Waldenström macroglobulinaemia

This disorder usually behaves in a low-grade fashion. Like CLL, this is a disease typically found in patients who are in their sixth or seventh decade. The malignant cells are mature B cells capable of secreting IgM. At a molecular level, acquired mutations in the *MYD88* gene are found in >90% of patients with this lymphoma entity, reflecting aberrant activation of the NF-κB intracellular signalling pathway in its pathogenesis. The bone marrow is typically involved, and lymphadenopathy is also a common feature.

Where IgM is secreted by the neoplastic cells, the disorder may be dominated by clinical manifestations of viscosity consequent on high levels of paraprotein; the condition is then known as Waldenström macroglobulinaemia. Hyperviscosity may cause headaches, visual disturbances (fundoscopic examination may reveal dilated veins, papilloedema and retinal haemorrhage) and altered consciousness. There may also be bleeding or thrombosis.

The IgM paraprotein may have unusual physical properties such as causing red cell agglutination (cold agglutinins) or precipitating in cold temperatures (cryoglobulin).

Patients are frequently anaemic and experience symptoms of tiredness and fatigue. The fatigue is often out of proportion to the level of haemoglobin. Systemic symptoms such as fever, weight loss and night sweats may occur, particularly if the lymphoma undergoes high-grade transformation.

Laboratory findings are summarized in Box 9.3.

Treatment and prognosis

Asymptomatic patients without anaemia and with low-level paraproteins can be monitored. If treatment is required, first-line chemotherapy typically involves an alkylating agent with the monoclonal antibody rituximab. In frailer patients, less aggressive regimens may be used. The BTK inhibitor ibrutinib is also effective and is typically used second-line although it may be used upfront in some cases. Remissions may last for years. High-dose treatment with autologous stem cell rescue is occasionally used in young patients with an aggressive clinical course.

Hyperviscosity syndrome requires urgent plasma exchange. Rituximab may cause a transient increase in IgM ('IgM flare') and is often omitted in the first course of treatment for patients with a high paraprotein. Patients receiving rituximab require careful paraprotein monitoring.

The prognosis is typically measurable in several years, with long remission periods after treatment. A small proportion of patients may undergo high-grade transformation to DLBCL, which is more challenging to treat.

Mantle cell lymphoma

Mantle cell lymphoma is an aggressive lymphoma. This entity is more common in males and generally presents in older patients with a median age of 60 years. The malignant cells are thought to derive from cells of the mantle zone of the lymph node follicle (Figure 9.9a). The lymphoma cells are small to medium sized and, in common with CLL, express CD5. In contrast to CLL, mantle cell lymphoma does not express CD23 and there is a characteristic cytogenetic abnormality that is found in nearly all cases. This is the translocation between chromosome 11 and chromosome 14, t(11;14), which leads to the

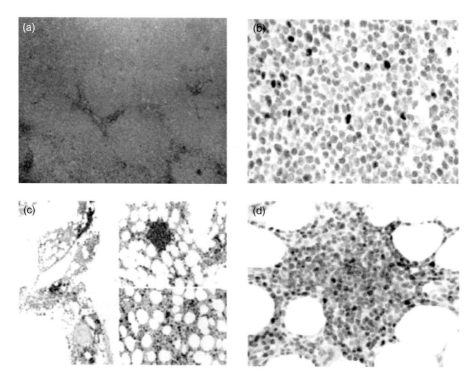

Figure 9.9 (a) The non-specific histological appearance seen in the biopsy of a patient with mantle cell lymphoma; (b) staining using an antibody against cyclin D1, which is overexpressed in mantle cell lymphoma; (c) minimal disease after treatment identified by cyclin D1 staining; (d) high-power view.

upregulation of the protein cyclin D1, known to have a key role in cell cycle regulation (Figure 9.9b). Mutations in *TP53* are associated with a poorer response to treatment. The immunophenotype is CD19+, CD20+, CD5+, CD23– and cyclin D1+.

Patients with the disorder present with widespread lymphadenopathy, hepatosplenomegaly and bone marrow involvement and in some cases abnormal lymphocytes can be seen in the peripheral blood. Some series have reported a very high incidence of gastrointestinal involvement (80%). Systemic symptoms are unusual, most patients feeling reasonably well at the time of presentation.

Treatment and prognosis

A minority of patients have indolent disease, characteristically those with a leukaemic presentation and low-volume lymphadenopathy. Such patients can be monitored. Involved field radiotherapy may be considered for those with stage I or localized stage II disease.

For the majority of fit patients requiring treatment at presentation, most centres offer combination chemotherapy, followed, assuming a response, by autologous stem cell transplant. At relapse, the BTK inhibitors (ibrutinib or acalabrutinib) are effective treatments and an allogeneic stem cell transplant may be considered in relapsed disease. CAR T-cell therapy with a CAR directed against CD19 also appears to lead to durable remissions at a similar rate, and is likely to be increasingly used in the future.

Mantle cell lymphoma is considered incurable with chemotherapy alone and has historically been very difficult to treat. With modern front-line intensive treatment, around 70–80% of patients will be alive at 5 years. Allogeneic stem cell transplant is curative in about 40% of relapsed patients but carries significant toxicity. CAR T-cell therapy holds considerable promise, although long-term efficacy data are awaited.

Hairy cell leukaemia

This uncommon low-grade lymphoproliferative disease frequently affects middle-aged males. Patients typically present with pancytopenia and splenomegaly. Characteristic 'hairy' cells are usually found on examination of a peripheral blood film (Figure 9.10). The disorder may be therefore suspected on microscopy of the blood and bone marrow, and diagnosis is assisted

by immunophenotyping. The immunophenotype is CD20+, CD5–, sIg+, CD25+, CD103+ and CD11c+. However, at a molecular level, this entity is now defined by a substitution (V600E) in the *BRAF* gene, which results in activation of the RAF-MEK-extracellular signal-regulated kinase (MEK-ERK) signalling cascade.

Hairy cell leukaemia responds well to treatment with purine analogue chemotherapy such as 2-chlorodeoxyadenosine (cladribine) or pentostatin, with long remissions typically lasting several years.

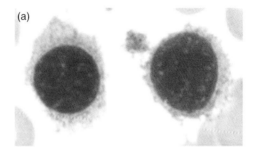

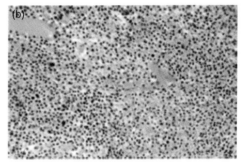

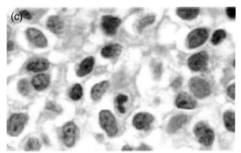

Figure 9.10 (a) Photomicrograph showing hairy cells in peripheral blood; (b) low-power view of trephine biopsy showing infiltration and haemorrhage; (c) high-power view of trephine biopsy. The hairy cells have bean-shaped nuclei and abundant clear cytoplasm (appearing like a halo around the nucleus).

These may be combined with rituximab at relapse. The monoclonal *BRAF* inhibitor vemurafenib has also been used therapeutically. The prognosis is excellent for most patients.

Extranodal marginal zone lymphomas, including the group previously known as MALT lymphomas

The mucosa-associated lymphoid tissue (MALT) lymphomas are typically extranodal, as their name suggests. This type of lymphoma belongs to the group of marginal zone lymphomas, as the malignant cells are thought to derive from the marginal zone of the lymphoid follicle. The most common type is gastric MALT lymphoma. Patients usually present with a long history of indigestion and are found to have MALT lymphoma on gastric biopsy. Some, but by no means all, are associated with the presence of *Helicobacter pylori*. Eradication of the bacterium using combination antibiotic therapy often leads to eradication of the lymphoma. In those cases that cannot be treated successfully with antibiotics, gentle oral chemotherapy or involved field radiotherapy will usually control the disease. High-grade transformation may occur and is treated in the usual way with combination chemotherapy. Other common sites involved with this lymphoma include the thyroid gland, salivary glands, lungs and spleen.

The immunophenotype is CD20+, CD79+, CD5-, CD23-, CD10- and sIgM+.

HIV-related lymphoma

The risk of developing HIV-related lymphoma is strongly linked to low CD4 counts and is considerably reduced with the introduction of highly active antiretroviral therapy (HAART). The most common lymphoma associated with HIV is DLBCL followed by Burkitt lymphoma, though Hodgkin lymphoma is also increased. The outcome for patients with HIV-associated lymphoma is greatly improved with the concomitant administration of antiretroviral treatment and standard immunochemotherapy.

The T-cell lymphomas

The mature or peripheral (as opposed to cutaneous) T-cell lymphomas are a heterogeneous group of disorders arising from clonal proliferation of post-thymic lymphocytes. In the Western world, they are significantly less common than B-cell malignancies. They usually have a CD4+ phenotype. Several variants are recognized, but a knowledge of all of these is only necessary for specialists – a brief summary of the most common is provided in Table 9.1.

Table 9.1 **The most common T-cell lymphomas.**

T-cell lymphoma	Clinical features
Peripheral T-cell lymphoma (unspecified)	Lymphadenopathy +/− marrow involvement. Generally poor prognosis
Angioimmunoblastic	Older patients, lymphadenopathy, rashes, fever; may see autoimmune manifestations
Anaplastic large cell lymphoma	Aggressive course, characterized by systemic symptoms and extranodal involvement. More prevalent in children. t(2;5)(p23;q35) which leads to overexpression of ALK. CD30+ neoplastic cells targeted for treatment by anti-CD30 antibody–drug conjugate
Adult T-cell leukaemia/ lymphoma (ATLL)	Caused by the human T-cell leukaemia/lymphoma virus type 1 (HTLV-1), endemic in parts of Japan and the Caribbean. Acute presentation with hypercalcaemia, skin lesions and lymphadenopathy. Treated with combination chemotherapy and antivirals
T-cell prolymphocytic leukaemia	Poor prognosis lymphoma typically presenting with splenomegaly and characteristically abnormal lymphocytes in the peripheral blood. Treated with the anti-CD52 antibody alemtuzumab
T-cell large granular lymphocytic leukaemia (T-LGL)	Typically presents with neutropenia (or other cytopenias), and may be associated with rheumatoid arthritis. May be treated with low-dose methotrexate
Mycosis fungoides and Sezary syndrome	T-cell lymphomas of the skin; usually require specialist dermatological input to guide treatment

Box 9.4 **Haematological emergency – tumour lysis syndrome**

Tumour lysis syndrome (TLS) is a constellation of metabolic abnormalities which results from chemotherapy- or radiotherapy-induced cell death. Occasionally it may occur spontaneously in very rapidly growing malignancies. Tumour cytotoxicity releases intracellular contents including nucleic acids, proteins and electrolytes into the circulation. Biochemically, this manifests as hyperuricaemia, hyperphosphataemia, hypocalcaemia and hyperkalaemia, with accompanying acute kidney injury. Clinically, patients may become anuric and develop life-threatening cardiac arrhythmias or seizures. Patients develop acute kidney injury due to the precipitation of urate crystals and/or calcium phosphate in the renal tubules. Without appropriate prophylaxis and recognition, morbidity and mortality are high.

Risk factors for development of TLS include:

- high-grade malignancies
- large tumour burden (manifesting as bulky lymphadenopathy and/or a markedly raised white cell count)
- pre-existing renal impairment
- increased age
- the use of particularly potent chemotherapy agents (for example, venetoclax)
- concomitant use of drugs which increase the uric acid level.

Tumour lysis syndrome is defined as two or more of the following.

Uric acid	≥476 micromol/L or 25% increase from baseline
Oliguria	Despite adequate hydration
Potassium*	≥6 mmol/L or 25% increase from baseline
Calcium	≤1.75 mmol/L or 25% decrease from baseline
Phosphate	≥1.45 mmol/L or 25% increase from baseline

For *clinical tumour lysis*, patient must have laboratory features, together with one of creatinine ≥1.5 × upper limit of normal, arrhythmia, seizure or sudden death. Conditions which are high risk for tumour lysis include:

- Burkitt lymphoma
- acute lymphoblastic leukaemia with a white cell count >100 × 10^9/L
- acute myeloid leukaemia with a WCC >100 × 10^9/L
- high-grade lymphoma with bulky disease defined as LDH 2× upper limit of normal or >10 cm lymphadenopathy.

Low/intermediate-risk patients can be managed with intravenous hydration and allopurinol – a xanthine oxidase inhibitor which blocks the conversion of purines to uric acid. For patients at high risk of or with established tumour lysis syndrome, rasburicase is used, both for prophylaxis and treatment. This is a recombinant urate oxidase derived from *Aspergillus*. All patients require frequent biochemical monitoring (up to every 6 h) with close monitoring of urine output and at least daily monitoring of weight.

It is important to note that even with rasburicase prophylaxis, tumour lysis syndrome still occurs in 5% of high-risk adult patients and 1.5% of high-risk paediatric patients. Whilst hyperkalaemia and hyperphosphataemia can in theory be managed medically, patients with established tumour lysis syndrome may require renal replacement therapy to avoid life-threatening complications. Prompt liaison with renal/critical care teams is essential.

10

Plasma cell myeloma and other paraproteinaemias

LEARNING OBJECTIVES

After reading this chapter, you should be able to:

✔ define the term 'paraprotein' and appreciate its clinical significance, including the common condition MGUS

✔ describe the pathology, clinical features and diagnosis of myeloma and understand the principles of treatment of this disorder

✔ suggest other important disorders which can be associated with paraproteins.

Plasma cell myeloma

Myeloma is a disease arising from the malignant transformation of a terminally differentiated B cell (plasma cell). The differentiating cells of the malignant clone have the morphology of plasma cells or plasmacytoid lymphocytes, have clonally rearranged immunoglobulin genes (see Chapter 1) and usually secrete a monoclonal immunoglobulin (IgG or IgA, very rarely IgM, IgD or IgE), a monoclonal light chain (κ or λ), or both.

Such monoclonal proteins are called paraproteins; they consist of structurally identical molecules and therefore produce a discrete monoclonal band (called an M band) on serum protein electrophoresis. As well as clones secreting intact immunoglobulins, approximately 20% of plasma cell clones secrete light chains only without a detectable paraprotein – this is called light chain myeloma.

The primary site of proliferation of the malignant plasma cells is the bone marrow. Activation of osteoclasts by molecules secreted from stromal cells and from the myeloma cells themselves causes bone destruction that leads to multiple well-defined osteolytic lesions and hypercalcaemia. Marrow infiltration also causes impairment of haematopoiesis. Some patients with IgA paraproteins (which dimerize) and a few patients with high levels of IgG3 paraproteins have a substantially raised plasma viscosity and may develop hyperviscosity syndrome.

Light chains are filtered through the glomeruli and are found in the urine; when they are present in excess, they may damage the renal tubules, in some cases leading to dialysis-dependent renal failure. In 10% of patients, the abnormally folded paraprotein is converted into deposits of amyloid in various tissues. Levels of normal immunoglobulin are reduced (referred to as immunoparesis) and in advanced disease there is a reduction in circulating T cells. Extramedullary tumour deposits of plasma cells may develop, particularly in advanced or aggressive disease.

Haematology Lecture Notes, Eleventh Edition. Deborah Hay, Andrew King and Michael Desborough.
© 2023 John Wiley & Sons Ltd. Published 2023 by John Wiley & Sons Ltd.
Companion website: www.wiley.com/go/Hay/Haematology/11e

How does myeloma develop? MGUS and smouldering/asymptomatic multiple myeloma

It is now well recognized that myeloma is always preceded by an asymptomatic phase in which a detectable paraprotein or excess of light chains is present without end-organ damage. The finding of a detectable paraprotein in an unselected population is common, being present in the serum of ~5% of over-50s, with an increasing incidence in the elderly. The majority of such individuals have a condition termed monoclonal gammopathy of undetermined significance (MGUS) which does not require treatment. By definition, patients with MGUS must have only a small population of clonal plasma cells (<10% on a bone marrow biopsy – though a biopsy is not needed in the majority of otherwise well patients with MGUS), and their paraprotein level is also low (<30g/L) with no evidence of end-organ damage arising as a result of these abnormalities.

The risk of MGUS transforming to a condition requiring treatment (typically myeloma; rarely other lymphoproliferative disorders) is approximately 1% annually. Patients with a paraprotein >15g/L, an IgA paraprotein or an abnormal serum free light chain ratio (a significant skew between κ and λ light chain synthesis) have a higher risk of transformation. The risk of progression to myeloma is monitored, usually in a primary care setting, with regular paraprotein estimations and blood counts.

The small plasma cell clone responsible for MGUS will expand over time. Once it reaches a threshold level (a paraprotein level of >30g/L or plasma cell population in the marrow of >10%), it is recognized that the likelihood of developing symptoms is increased. This marks the transition from MGUS to 'smouldering' or asymptomatic myeloma, a condition in which the risk of transforming to symptomatic myeloma rises to approximately 10% per year. The monitoring of such patients is then transferred to haematologists, and clinical trials are ongoing to assess whether treatment prior to development of end-organ damage is beneficial.

The diagnosis of symptomatic myeloma usually requires evidence of end-organ damage, commonly remembered as the CRAB criteria:

- hyper**C**alcaemia (>2.75 mmol/L or >0.25 mmol/L higher than upper limit of normal)
- **R**enal impairment (serum creatinine >177 μmol/L or creatinine clearance <40 mL/min)
- **A**naemia (Hb <100 g/L or 20 g/L below lower limit of normal)
- **B**one lesions – one or more lytic bone lesion >5 mm on CT or PET-CT.

In rare cases where the marrow plasma cell percentage is >60% or the light chain ratio is very markedly skewed without end-organ damage, symptomatic myeloma may still be diagnosed.

The diagnostic criteria for MGUS, smouldering myeloma and symptomatic myeloma are summarised in Table 10.1.

Epidemiology

The age-standardized incidence of myeloma is about 40 per million of the population per year. With an ageing population, approximately 5800 new cases are diagnosed each year in the UK. Most patients are between the ages of 50 and 80 years with the median diagnosis being 66–70 years. Myeloma is twice as common in those with an Afro-Caribbean background and is slightly more common in men. Relatives of patients with MGUS or myeloma have a slightly higher relative risk of developing MGUS and myeloma (about three-fold) than the general population.

Table 10.1 Diagnostic criteria for monoclonal gammopathy of undetermined significance (MGUS), smouldering myeloma and plasma cell myeloma.

MGUS	Smouldering myeloma	Plasma cell myeloma
All three criteria must be met: 1 Serum M-protein (non-IgM) <30g/L 2 Clonal bone marrow plasma cells <10% 3 Absence of end-organ damage that can be attributed to the plasma cell proliferative disorder	Both criteria must be met: 1 Serum M-protein (IgG or IgA) ≥30g/L or urinary M-protein >500mg/24 h and/or clonal bone marrow plasma cells 10–60% 2 Absence of myeloma-defining events or amyloidosis	Both criteria must be met: 1 Clonal bone marrow plasma cells ≥10% or biopsy proven plasmacytoma 2 One or more myeloma-defining events

Clinical features

Bone destruction

The most common presenting symptom is bone pain, typically over the lumbar spine. Pathological fractures and lytic lesions are frequent and often affect the lower thoracic and upper lumbar vertebrae, the ribs, pelvis and long bones (humeri and femora). Lytic lesions may also be seen within the skull, giving a 'raindrop' appearance (Figure 10.1).

Previously, plain films were used to assess for bony damage but these are less sensitive than whole-body CT or MRI, which most centres now routinely use for patient assessment. Compression fractures of the vertebrae may damage the spinal cord or spinal roots and cause neurological symptoms. Collections of plasma cells may form in relation to any bone (a plasmacytoma) and cause pressure symptoms, including spinal cord compression (Figure 10.2 and Box 10.1).

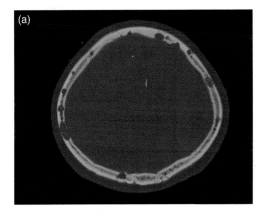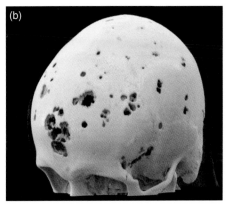

Figure 10.1 (a) Transverse low-dose CT of the skull showing lytic lesions in myeloma. (b) A 3D reconstruction shows the 'raindrop' skull appearance.
Source: Courtesy of Dr Timothy Sadler, Cambridge University Hospitals NHS Foundation Trust.

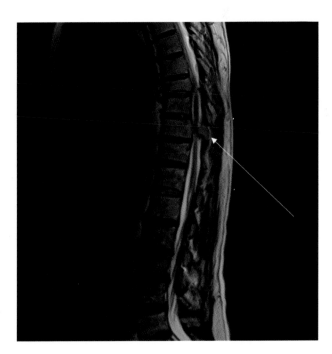

Figure 10.2 MRI of the spine showing spinal cord compression (indicated by arrow) secondary to myeloma. Disease can also be seen throughout the vertebral column.
Source: Courtesy of Dr Timothy Sadler, Cambridge University Hospitals NHS Foundation Trust.

> **Box 10.1 Haematological emergency – spinal cord compression**
>
> Spinal cord compression may occur in haematological malignancies due to tumour within the cord, spinal dura or meninges, extension of a vertebral tumour into the spinal canal or vertebral collapse with retropulsion of a bony fragment into the spinal cord.
>
> Spinal cord compression in haematological malignancies is most common in myeloma (up to 20% of patients) but can also be seen in Hodgkin lymphoma and non-Hodgkin lymphoma.
>
> Patients typically report back pain (although 15% of patients may have no or minimal pain) which is characteristically worse at night. Weakness is common, with patients often saying an extremity is weak or clumsy. Around 70% of patients are unable to walk at diagnosis. Patients may also report sensory disturbance. Autonomic symptoms including urinary retention and faecal incontinence are late signs and their absence should not be used to exclude spinal cord compression.
>
> The diagnostic investigation of choice is an MRI of the whole spine, which should be performed urgently within 24 hours of presentation. It is important to image the whole spine rather than attempt to use examination to rationalize imaging as up to 40% of patients may have multiple levels of impingement.
>
> Following diagnosis, treatment should be instigated without delay and includes high-dose dexamethasone (typically 20–40 mg once daily in myeloma for 4 days) and evaluation for a decompressive surgical procedure by a spinal surgeon. In patients deemed unsuitable for surgery (due to poor performance status or prognosis), radiotherapy forms the mainstay of treatment. Systemic treatment may be initiated as soon as practical following recovery from surgery.

Renal failure

Acute kidney injury may be found at presentation in patients with a high light chain burden, or may develop during the course of the disease. Chronic renal failure commonly results from the obstruction of distal renal tubules by proteinaceous casts, leading to tubular atrophy and interstitial fibrosis (myeloma kidney). Renal dysfunction may also result from the toxic effects of light chains on tubule cells, the deposition of light chains in glomeruli and, more rarely, amyloidosis. Acute kidney injury may be precipitated by dehydration, use of analgesics such as non-steroidal anti-inflammatory drugs, sepsis, hypercalcaemia or hyperuricaemia.

Bone marrow failure

Anaemia is common in myeloma and is usually normocytic or mildly macrocytic. Paraproteins may interfere with fibrin polymerization or platelet function, although significant bleeding symptoms at presentation are rare. Neutropenia and thrombocytopenia may develop in advanced cases.

Bacterial infections

Respiratory tract infections are common in patients with myeloma. The lack of normal antibodies (acquired hypogammaglobulinaemia) results in infections caused by encapsulated organisms, commonly *Streptococcus pneumoniae* and *Haemophilus influenzae*.

Hypercalcaemia

Hypercalcaemia causes symptoms such as anorexia, vomiting, lethargy, stupor and coma, or patients may present more acutely with polyuria and polydipsia (see Box 10.2).

Hyperviscosity syndrome

This is characterized by neurological disturbances (dizziness, somnolence and coma), cardiac failure and haemorrhagic manifestations (Figure 10.3). IgA myeloma is more likely to cause hyperviscosity, as IgA has a tendency to form dimers. The very rare IgM myeloma is also associated with hyperviscosity given that IgM forms pentamers (IgM paraproteins usually suggest lymphoplasmacytic lymphoma, however, see Chapter 9). It is uncommon for IgG myeloma patients to have hyperviscosity unless the paraprotein is very high (often >70 g/L); it is somewhat more common with the IgG3 subtype, the paraprotein of which has a tendency to aggregate. Hyperviscosity syndrome is treated by emergency plasma exchange along with prompt initiation of anti-myeloma therapy.

Laboratory findings

A normochromic normocytic or macrocytic anaemia is common. When the disease is advanced, thrombocytopenia and neutropenia may also be found. The blood film may show a leucoerythroblastic picture (reflecting marrow infiltration) and, in occasional

Box 10.2 **Haematological emergency – hypercalcaemia**

Symptoms of hypercalcaemia include:

- polyuria and polydipsia
- constipation
- abdominal pain and vomiting
- tiredness, weakness and confusion
- in severe cases – coma.

Potential causative medications including thiazide diuretics, vitamin D supplements and calcium supplements should be stopped and other causes considered, including primary hyperparathyroidism.

Mild hypercalcaemia (2.60–3.0 mmol/L) can be managed with oral hydration and rarely requires admission. IV bisphosphonates may be given on an outpatient basis.

Moderate hypercalcaemia (3.0–3.4 mmol/L) may require admission dependent upon

symptoms and other blood tests (for example, renal function).

Severe hypercalcaemia (>3.4 mmol/L) requires admission for management.

Moderate hypercalcaemia with symptoms or severe hypercalcaemia may be managed as follows.

- Rehydration with IV 0.9% saline, to correct volume depletion from calcium-induced diuresis and decreased fluid intake and also to promote renal calcium excretion. Calcium can be expected to drop by approximately 0.25 mmol/L.

- An IV bisphosphonate (e.g. zoledronic acid) should be given 24–48 hours after rehydration. This normally corrects hypercalcaemia in 5–8 days.

- In myeloma, steroids are usually started in addition and definitive chemotherapy when practical.

- In refractory cases, additional treatments may be required, including calcitonin.

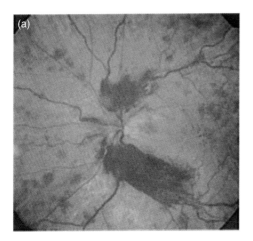
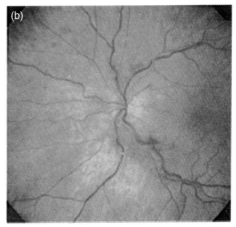

Figure 10.3 Fundi of the eyes in the hyperviscosity syndrome showing (a) retinal haemorrhages and (b) papilloedema.

patients, circulating plasma cells may be present. Red cells may form rouleaux (Figure 10.4), which reflects changes to the rheology of the blood caused by the high protein level. The paraprotein may cause an increased basophilic staining of the background between the red cells. The erythrocyte sedimentation rate (ESR) is often raised, frequently to more than 100 mm/h. The serum uric acid is raised in about half of cases (and may therefore contribute to the renal damage).

Free light chains are detected in the serum using the sensitive serum free light chain (SFLC) immunoassay. Under normal circumstances, the κ:λ ratio is 0.26–1.65 and this becomes skewed when there is an excess of light chains (often the free κ or λ can measure in the 1000s). The κ:λ ratio may also be skewed in chronic kidney disease due to greater retention of κ light chains (normal range changing to 0.37–3) and both κ and λ light chains may be increased in infection. It is therefore important to interpret

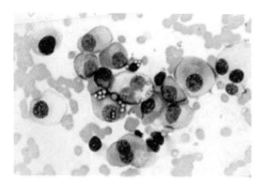

Figure 10.5 A marrow smear from a patient with multiple myeloma. MGG stain.

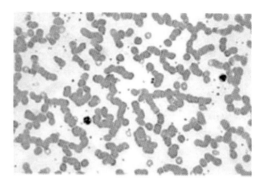

Figure 10.4 Blood film from a patient with plasma cell myeloma showing marked red cell rouleau formation. MGG stain.

SFLC results in the clinical context of the patient. Free light chains may separately be detected using urine electrophoresis (also called Bence-Jones proteins when present in the urine).

In 1–2% of patients with myeloma, a paraprotein cannot be detected in serum and light chains cannot be detected in concentrated urine: this is termed non-secretory myeloma and can present a challenge to diagnosis. It should be considered in patients with clinical features suggestive of myeloma and a general reduction in immunoglobulin levels.

Bone marrow aspirates in myeloma usually contain a greatly increased proportion of plasma cells (Figure 10.5). Some aspirates may show only a slight increase in plasma cells (5–10% of nucleated marrow cells, compared with 0.1–2% in normal marrow). The latter results from the multifocal nature of the plasma cell infiltrate. Bone marrow trephines may provide a more accurate assessment of proportion of plasma cells and both an aspirate and trephine should be performed at diagnosis.

Because myeloma is typically present throughout the bone marrow at diagnosis, conventional staging (as performed in lymphoma) is unhelpful. Patients are therefore 'staged' for prognostic purposes using the Revised Multiple Myeloma International Staging System (R-ISS). Patients whose malignant plasma cells harbour certain abnormalities such as t(4;14), del 17p (which contains the gene *TP53*) or t(14;16) are at higher risk of progression and have shorter overall survival. These results are combined with the serum lactate dehydrogenase (LDH), serum albumin and serum β_2-microglobulin, allowing separation into three groups (Figure 10.6).

R-ISS staging for plasma cell myeloma

Stage	Laboratory features	Approx overall survival at 5 years
Stage I	All of the following criteria are met: • Serum beta-2 microglobulin < 3.5 mg/L • Normal serum albumin • Normal serum lactate dehydrogenase • Cytogenetic studies show no 'high risk' changes	~80%
Stage II	Does not meet criteria for either stage I or stage III	~60%
Stage III	Raised serum beta-2 microglobulin (>5.5 mg/L) and one of the following: • Cytogenetic studies showing 'high risk' changes • Raised serum LDH	~40%

Figure 10.6 The R-ISS staging system with survival shown for each group.

(a)

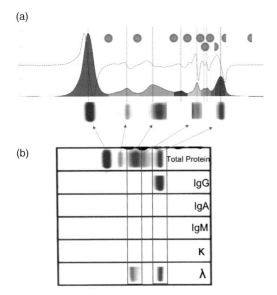

(b)

				Total Protein
				IgG
				IgA
				IgM
				K
				λ

Figure 10.7 Myeloma screening investigations.
(a) Initial screening performed by capillary zone electrophoresis on serum. Here there are abnormal peaks in the protein spectrum, particularly in the 'gamma' region of the serum (hatched orange peak, far right) and the 'alpha-2' region (light orange zone, 3rd from left). (b) These abnormal peaks are then further investigated by serum immunofixation on gel. This confirms a monoclonal IgG λ paraprotein in the gamma region, and a free λ light chain in the alpha-2 region.
Source: Courtesy of Dr Ross Sadler, Oxford University Hospitals NHS Foundation Trust.

Electrophoresis of serum usually demonstrates the monoclonal Ig as a discrete band (M band; Figure 10.7). The nature of the paraprotein can be determined by immunofixation. In 50% of patients with myeloma, the paraprotein is IgG, in 25% it is IgA, in 20% it is light chain only, and in 1–2% it is IgD or IgE. IgM-producing myelomas are extremely rare.

Treatment

Treatment requires a multidisciplinary approach involving haematologists, radiation oncologists and specialist nurses.

Supportive care

Supportive care measures are very important. Anaemia is a common finding at presentation or progression and may also arise due to treatment.

Patients who require frequent transfusion may benefit from subcutaneous erythropoietin. Adequate hydration must be maintained in an attempt to reduce the risk of paraprotein precipitation in the renal tubules and consequent renal damage. Haemodialysis is required in the event of renal failure. Bacterial infections, caused by the associated acquired hypogammaglobulinaemia, require prompt treatment with antibiotics. There is good evidence that prophylactic antibiotics (levofloxacin) during induction treatment decrease mortality. Prophylactic infusions of immunoglobulin concentrates may be considered in patients with recurrent infections. Hyperviscosity syndrome may be treated with plasma exchange. Bone pain and fractures and hypercalcaemia cause significant morbidity and mortality in patients with myeloma, and long-term therapy with bisphosphonates (such as zoledronic acid) has been shown to reduce bone pain and progression of skeletal lesions. Orthopaedic surgery may be required for critical lytic lesions.

Chemotherapy

Stratification of patients according to their outcome risk (see above), their eligibility for high-dose therapy (based on age, performance status, etc.) and the funding arrangements in place in the treating country dictates the chemotherapy management strategy employed.

There is excellent evidence to support the use of high-dose chemotherapy and peripheral stem cell rescue (see Chapter 12) as first-line treatment in younger (<75 years), fit patients with myeloma. For those patients who are transplant eligible, initial treatment begins with combination induction chemotherapy typically incorporating a proteasome inhibitor such as bortezomib (Velcade®) together with an immunomodulatory drug (IMiD) such as thalidomide or lenalidomide with dexamethasone. The treatment is consolidated in responding patients with autologous bone marrow transplantation using high-dose melphalan as conditioning, and then typically followed by maintenance treatment with lenalidomide until progression. CD38 antibody-directed therapy (daratumumab) may be used during induction in high-risk patients and is an important therapy at relapse.

The duration of remission may be long (>5 years) in those patients fit enough to receive high-dose therapy followed by maintenance. Patients unable to receive high-dose therapy because of comorbidities are usually treated with similar induction regimens, and response rates are usually high (>80%). Careful management of adverse effects of chemotherapy, whether related to marrow suppression, neurological dysfunction or thromboembolism, is essential.

However, myeloma is conventionally considered incurable and the vast majority of patients (>90%) will eventually relapse, requiring retreatment. The treatment landscape for myeloma continues to evolve rapidly, with bispecific antibodies (which bring T cells together with myeloma cells as a form of immunotherapy) and CAR T cells directed against myeloma-specific antigens in late-phase clinical trials. It is likely both will become standard therapies in the next few years.

Radiotherapy

Radiotherapy is a very effective treatment for bone pain in myeloma. Spinal cord compression caused by a vertebral or paravertebral mass requires urgent assessment, and decompression laminectomy followed by radiotherapy is usually the treatment of choice. Bone fractures, a common complication, are best treated by orthopaedic fixation followed by radiotherapy. Painful lytic lesions respond well to single fractions of palliative radiotherapy, usually with minimal side-effects.

Other paraproteinaemias and related disorders

Solitary plasmacytoma

Solitary tumours consisting of a single mass of clonal plasma cells may be found arising from bones (intraosseous) or in extramedullary sites such as the upper respiratory or gastrointestinal tracts. It is common to find a paraprotein in the serum and/or an increase in free κ or λ. Full staging, typically with PET-CT and bone marrow biopsy, is necessary prior to therapy to exclude the presence of additional sites of disease. Treatment typically consists of radical radiotherapy; surgery may also be performed prior to radiotherapy in certain cases (for example, in spinal instability). Patients require monitoring following treatment as there is a relatively high rate of progression to plasma cell myeloma (as high as 80% at 10 years for some solitary bone plasmacytomas; the risk is lower for extramedullary plasmacytomas).

Plasma cell leukaemia

This rare disease is defined by a high number of circulating plasma cells in the peripheral blood (>5% of white cells). Clinically, patients will often have a pancytopenia and organomegaly in conjunction with features found in myeloma (hypercalcaemia, lytic lesions and renal impairment). The plasma cells typically harbour cytogenetic findings associated with high-risk myeloma in addition to t(11;14). It is treated with myeloma-directed therapy; responses tend to be short and prognosis is poor.

Amyloidosis

Amyloidosis is a heterogeneous group of disorders of protein folding whereby normally soluble proteins are deposited as β-pleated sheets. Infiltration of organs with amyloid leads to dysfunction and eventual organ failure. Amyloid may be demonstrated in bone marrow, rectal, gingival, subcutaneous fat or renal biopsies; it stains positively with Congo red and shows an apple-green birefringence in polarized light (Figure 10.8). Amyloid may be one of three principal types, only one of which is related to an abnormal plasma cell clone.

- *AA amyloid.* This is seen in patients with long-term chronic infections or inflammatory disorders (for example, rheumatoid arthritis). The amyloid protein is derived from serum amyloid A-related protein. This protein is synthesized in inflammatory states and, if present for long enough at a high enough level, becomes deposited in various organs. Treatment is directed at the underlying condition. It is not related to the plasma cell disorders.
- *AL amyloid.* These proteins consist of part or all of the immunoglobulin light chain. The classic features include macroglossia, carpal tunnel syndrome, peripheral neuropathy (all related to amyloid deposition) and purpura (due to dysfunction of clotting factors bound by amyloid protein), but more important clinically are malabsorption, nephrotic syndrome and a restrictive cardiomyopathy. Patients are found to have raised κ or λ light chains, with raised λ light chains being more common. AL amyloid may be found in patients with <10% plasma cells in the marrow or in patients with symptomatic myeloma. Patients with cardiac involvement have a poor prognosis (often <6 months). Treatment is directed at the plasma cell clone and a minority of patients will also be fit

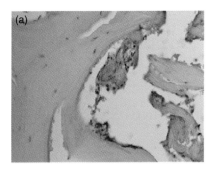 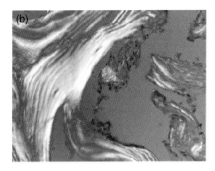

Figure 10.8 (a) A bone marrow biopsy showing an AL amyloid deposit in the blood vessel staining with Congo red. (b) Polarized light shows the typical apple-green birefringence.
Source: Courtesy of Dr Pedro Martin Cabrera, Cambridge University Hospitals NHS Foundation Trust.

enough to undergo high-dose treatment with autologous stem cell rescue.

- *Familial forms.* This is a diverse group of diseases, often presenting as neuropathy but frequently involving other organs, including the heart. The most common is due to mutations in transthyretin. Several treatments, including gene therapy, are in development but are not yet routinely available. They are not related to plasma cell disorders.

POEMS syndrome

This rare and interesting disorder, also called osteosclerotic myeloma, is characterized by a paraprotein (almost always λ restricted) associated with a variety of paraneoplastic phenomena including a demyelinating polyneuropathy, osteosclerotic bone lesions, organomegaly (for example, hepatomegaly or splenomegaly), an endocrinopathy (for example, hypoadrenalism or hypothyroidism) and skin changes. Treatment may involve radiotherapy if disease is localized or systemic chemotherapy treatment if there is marrow involvement. Patients in the latter group who are well enough to undergo autologous stem cell transplant often have a significant clinical improvement.

Waldenström macroglobulinaemia

Waldenström macroglobulinaemia (or lymphoplasmacytic lymphoma; see Chapter 9 for greater detail) is also characterized by the presence of a paraprotein, although, in contrast to myeloma, in this condition it is nearly always IgM. The IgM paraprotein is secreted by a clonal population of pleomorphic lymphocytes and plasma cells that infiltrate the bone marrow, lymph nodes and spleen. Symptoms result from both tissue infiltration and hyperviscosity of the blood caused by high levels of IgM. Osteolytic lesions are rare. It is a relatively uncommon condition, being found at approximately 10% of the incidence of myeloma.

Heavy chain diseases

In these rare paraproteinaemias, the B-lineage-derived malignant clone secretes γ, α or μ heavy chains rather than complete immunoglobulin molecules. The clinical picture is that of a lymphoma; α-chain disease is characterized by severe malabsorption caused by infiltration of the small intestine by lymphoma cells. Treatment is normally lymphoma based directed against the B-cell clone.

Other lymphoproliferative disorders

A paraprotein may also be found in chronic cold haemagglutinin disease in some patients with other types of non-Hodgkin lymphoma and chronic lymphocytic leukaemia. Such patients typically have low-level paraproteins.

11

Aplastic anaemia and pure red cell aplasia

LEARNING OBJECTIVES

After reading this chapter, you should be able to:

✓ describe the possible aetiologies of acquired aplastic anaemia, including the inherited causes

✓ outline the clinical and laboratory features, natural history and principles of treatment of acquired aplastic anaemia

✓ describe the clinical features of pure red cell aplasia and its possible aetiologies.

Aplastic anaemia

Aplastic anaemia is a disorder characterized by pancytopenia (i.e. a reduction in the number of red cells, neutrophils and platelets in the peripheral blood) with a marked decrease in the amount of haematopoietic tissue in the bone marrow (i.e. marrow aplasia or hypoplasia) and the absence of evidence of involvement of the marrow by diseases such as leukaemia, myeloma or carcinoma. The causes of aplastic anaemia are summarized in Box 11.1.

Acquired aplastic anaemia

This is an uncommon disease, the prevalence in Europe being between 1 and 3 per 100,000 people. It affects all ages with two peaks, one in adolescents and young adults and the other in people over the age of 60 years.

Box 11.1 Causes of aplastic anaemia

Inherited
- Fanconi anaemia
- Dyskeratosis congenita

Acquired
- Idiopathic (accounts for 70–80% of cases)
- Drugs and chemicals:
  - Dose dependent: cytotoxic drugs, benzene
  - Idiosyncratic: chloramphenicol, non-steroidal anti-inflammatory drugs
- Radiation
- Viruses: hepatitis viruses, Epstein–Barr virus, HIV
- Autoimmune disease (systemic lupus erythematosus)

Aplastic anaemia may also develop after a single large dose of whole-body irradiation (for example, as seen following the atomic bomb explosions in Hiroshima and Nagaskai, or in radiation accidents).

Haematology Lecture Notes, Eleventh Edition. Deborah Hay, Andrew King and Michael Desborough.
© 2023 John Wiley & Sons Ltd. Published 2023 by John Wiley & Sons Ltd.
Companion website: www.wiley.com/go/Hay/Haematology/11e

Aetiology

In 70–80% of cases no aetiological factors can be identified; such patients are described as having idiopathic acquired aplastic anaemia. The majority of other cases are due to inherited bone marrow failure syndromes. Rarely, aplasia is associated with exposure to specific drugs or chemicals, ionizing radiation or certain viruses including EBV and HIV. Hepatitis-associated aplastic anaemia accounts for 2–5% of cases in the West. This occurs most frequently in young males and characteristically develops 1–3 months after an acute episode of hepatitis. Testing for the known viral and autoimmune causes of hepatitis is typically negative; despite this, liver biopsies are normally consistent with an autoimmune hepatitis, and it is likely that the following aplastic anaemia is immune mediated.

Most cases of secondary aplastic anaemia result from an idiosyncratic reaction to the use of drugs. Many such drugs have been implicated, including phenylbutazone, indometacin, ibuprofen, sodium aurothiomalate, chloramphenicol, trimethoprim-sulfamethoxazole (co-trimoxazole) or organic arsenicals, anticonvulsants (phenytoin, carbamazepine) and antithyroid drugs (carbimazole, propylthiouracil). Some drugs predictably cause aplastic anaemia if given in sufficiently large doses: these include alkylating agents (e.g. busulfan, melphalan and cyclophosphamide), purine analogues and folate antagonists. Benzene is an example of an industrial chemical that often produces aplastic anaemia if inhaled in a sufficient dose; kerosene, carbon tetrachloride and insecticides such as DDT and chlordane can also cause aplasia of the marrow. A careful family history, drug history and occupational history of patients presenting with unexplained pancytopenia are mandatory.

Pathophysiology

The pancytopenia and marrow aplasia appear to be the consequence of damage to the multipotent haematopoietic stem cells, mediated by T cells, which impairs their self-renewal (see Chapter 1) and causes stem cell depletion.

The majority of cases of acquired idiopathic aplastic anaemia are autoimmune in pathophysiology. The T lymphocytes of some patients with acquired aplastic anaemia have been shown to inhibit the *in vitro* growth of haematopoietic colonies from autologous and allogeneic bone marrow.

This finding, together with the response of about 70% of patients to anti-thymocyte globulin (ATG) and ciclosporin, indicates that autoimmune mechanisms are involved in at least the persistence of the aplasia, if not its initiation.

Clinical features

Both idiopathic and secondary aplastic anaemia occur at all ages. The onset is often insidious. Symptoms include:

- lassitude, weakness and shortness of breath due to anaemia
- haemorrhagic manifestations resulting from the thrombocytopenia
- fever and recurrent infections as a consequence of neutropenia.

Haemorrhagic manifestations include epistaxis, bleeding from the gums, menorrhagia, bleeding into the gastrointestinal and urinary tracts, ecchymoses and petechiae. The severity of symptoms is variable and depends on the severity of the cytopenias. In patients with severe neutropenia and thrombocytopenia, fulminating infections (e.g. pneumonia) and cerebral haemorrhage are common causes of death. In secondary aplastic anaemia, symptoms may appear several weeks or months, or occasionally one or more years, after discontinuation of exposure to the causative drug or chemical. Splenomegaly is rare in aplastic anaemia and if this is present, alternative diagnoses should be explored.

Haematological findings

By definition, patients must have two of a haemoglobin <100 g/L, a platelet count <50 × 10^9/L, and a neutrophil count <1.5 × 10^9/L. The absolute reticulocyte count is low and is an important test. Some patients also have a reduced absolute lymphocyte count, although in most patients this remains normal. There is a marked increase in serum erythropoietin levels.

The bone marrow smear contains markedly hypocellular marrow fragments, with most of the volume of the fragments being made up of fat cells (Figure 11.1). Haematopoietic cells of all types, including megakaryocytes, are decreased or absent, and in severe aplastic anaemia the majority of the cells seen are plasma cells, lymphocytes, mast cells and macrophages. Residual erythropoietic cells may be morphologically abnormal. In order to obtain a

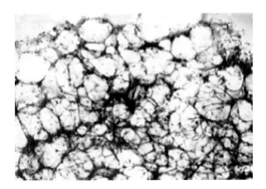

Figure 11.1 A bone marrow aspirate spicule from a patient with aplastic anaemia. The fragment is composed mostly of fat cells, with rather few haematopoietic cells.

reliable estimate of marrow cellularity, it is essential to examine histological sections of a trephine biopsy of the iliac crest (Figure 11.2). This not only provides a larger volume of marrow for study than a single marrow aspirate, but also helps exclude other causes of pancytopenia including foci of blasts suggesting an underlying hypoplastic leukaemia, dysplastic features or evidence of metastatic carcinoma. Marrow cellularity is normally <10% in severe aplastic anaemia.

Most patients have a normal karyotype at diagnosis. However, approximately 10% of patients have copy-number neutral loss of heterozygosity on chromosome 6p involving the human leucocyte antigen (HLA) locus, occurring due to selective pressure to escape immune surveillance through deletion of HLA alleles. Other cytogenetic abnormalites may also be seen, including monosomy 7, trisomy 8 and trisomy 6. Clonal haematopoiesis with somatic mutations of genes such as *PIGA*, *ASXL1* and *DNMT3A* is present in at least 50% of cases.

Approximately 50% of patients with acquired aplastic anaemia have a detectable PNH clone (see Chapter 3) and about 10% of patients have evidence of associated haemolysis.

Diagnosis

Other causes of pancytopenia (particularly leukaemia) should be considered and excluded before a diagnosis of aplastic anaemia is made. The causes of pancytopenia are summarized in Box 11.2. It is increasingly recognized that a proportion of patients with presumed idiopathic aplastic anaemia presenting in adulthood may have an inherited bone marrow failure syndrome (Box 11.3). It is therefore becoming routine practice to test all patients for inherited bone marrow failure syndromes using gene panels which contain the known mutated genes. This is particularly important when patients fail to respond to first-line immunosuppression or related donors are being considered for bone marrow transplantation.

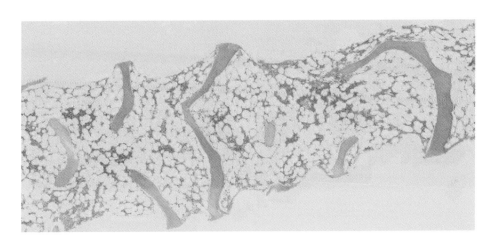

Figure 11.2 Section of a trephine biopsy of the bone marrow from a patient with aplastic anaemia showing marked hypocellularity. Haemotoxylin and eosin.

Box 11.2 Causes of pancytopenia

Mainly caused by a failure of production of cells
Bone marrow infiltration: leukaemia, myeloma, carcinoma, myelofibrosis, lipid storage disorders, osteopetrosis
Severe vitamin B12 or folate deficiency
Myelodysplastic syndromes
HIV infection
Aplastic anaemia
Anorexia nervosa

Mainly caused by an increased peripheral destruction of cells
Splenomegaly
Overwhelming infection
Systemic lupus erythematosus
Paroxysmal nocturnal haemoglobinuria[a]

[a]In some cases, there is also impaired production of cells because of hypoplasia of the marrow.

Treatment

If a causative drug or chemical is identified, exposure to this agent should be stopped. Supportive therapy including red cell transfusions, platelet transfusions, prophylactic antibiotics and antifungals is often required; the extent of supportive therapy depends on the degree of cytopenias. Neutropenic patients are at risk of overwhelming sepsis, and require admission for urgent intravenous antibiotic treatment if febrile. Platelet transfusions are indicated only in the context of haemorrhage or ATG treatment (which causes platelet consumption), as repeated platelet transfusions lead to alloimmunization and a reduction of the efficacy of subsequent platelet transfusions. Iron chelation may be necessary for heavily transfused patients.

The preferred treatment for idiopathic acquired aplastic anaemia depends upon the age of the patient, availability of an HLA-matched sibling and severity of the disease. Bone marrow transplantation is indicated at diagnosis for fit younger patients

Box 11.3 Inherited bone marrow failure syndromes

Fanconi anaemia
- A disorder of defective DNA repair. Inheritance is autosomal recessive. At least 16 different disease genes have been identified.

- Onset of pancytopenia between the ages of 5 and 10 years although some patients are diagnosed in their 40s or 50s.

- Frequent association with other congenital abnormalities (e.g. skin pigmentation, short stature, microcephaly, skeletal defects, genital hypoplasia and renal abnormalities).

- Various chromosomal abnormalities (breaks, rearrangements, exchanges and endoreduplications) in cultured lymphocytes exposed to diepoxybutane (DEB). This is used as a diagnostic test.

- Increased incidence of acute leukaemia (in 10% of patients) and solid tumours.

- Allogeneic bone marrow transplantation may cure the aplastic anaemia, but does not prevent the appearance of solid tumours. Conditioning regimes avoid radiotherapy given the increased risk of solid tumours.

Dyskeratosis congenita
- A disease of defective telomere maintenance. Can be inherited in an X-linked, autosomal dominant or autosomal recessive pattern. At least 10 genes have been identified.

- Characterized by a triad of abnormal skin pigmentation, nail dystrophy and oral leucoplakia in combination with bone marrow failure.

- Bone marrow failure occurs in 80–90% of patients by the age of 30. Pulmonary fibrosis and solid tumours are other complications.

- Allogeneic bone marrow transplantation may be curative.

Shwachman–Diamond syndrome
- A disorder of defective ribosome biogenesis, with mutations in the *SDBS* gene.

- Characterized by pancreatic insufficiency, bone marrow dysfunction (mainly neutropenia) and skeletal abnormalities.

- Patients have a predisposition to acute myeloid leukaemia and myelodysplasia.

- Management requires a multidisciplinary approach given the multisystem nature of the condition.

(less than 50 years) with severe or very severe aplastic anaemia if a HLA-matched sibling is available. Long-term survival is seen in >80% of cases. A specific concern is graft rejection, which occurs at a higher rate than in malignant conditions and may occur many months after transplantation. Children without an HLA-matched sibling may still proceed to transplant as first-line treatment if a well-matched unrelated donor is available.

Patients over the age of 50 or without an HLA-matched sibling are typically treated with immunosuppressive therapy comprising ATG and ciclosporin. Eltrombopag, a thrombopoietin agonist, has improved response rates in combination with ATG/ciclosporin to 70–80%. Response can take 3–6 months. Bone marrow transplant can be considered for fit patients who have failed first-line immunosuppressive therapy.

Antithymocyte globulin requires administration in an inpatient setting due to the risk of anaphylactic reactions. Serum sickness, a type III hypersensitivity reaction, may occur 7–21 days following administration, manifesting as a fever, joint pain, lymphadenopathy and proteinuria; prophylactic steroids are given for several days after treatment to reduce the risk of this.

The overall survival for patients with severe aplastic anaemia has improved considerably and is now greater than 70% at 5 years. However, relapse after ATG occurs in a proportion of patients; there is a risk of later clonal evolution to MDS/acute myeloid leukaemia and haemolytic PNH may develop in a minority of patients. Patients therefore require long-term follow-up.

Prognosis

Patients with both idiopathic and secondary acquired aplastic anaemia show a variable clinical course. About 15% of patients have a severe illness from the outset and die within 3 months of diagnosis, mainly due to infection.

Patients with the highest risk of complications are those with very severe aplastic anaemia, defined by a platelet count less than 20×10^9/L, a neutrophil count below 0.2×10^9/L, a reticulocyte count under 10×10^9/L and marked hypocellularity of the marrow. For patients who do not meet the criteria for severe disease, the prognosis of aplastic anaemia is relatively good. Even those with very severe cytopenias now have a much-improved prognosis compared with 10 or 20 years ago, largely due to improvements in treatment and supportive care.

Pure red cell aplasia

Rarely, aplasia or severe hypoplasia affects only the erythropoietic cells. Patients with this abnormality have a normochromic normocytic anaemia and reticulocytopenia with normal white cell and platelet counts.

The causes of pure red cell aplasia (PRCA) are listed in Box 11.4. In the rare congenital form, Diamond–Blackfan anaemia, clinical features usually develop in infancy and the haematological picture is associated with various congenital malformations, including craniofacial abnormalities and defects of the thumb and upper limbs. Genetic mutations involve genes encoding ribosomal proteins of small and large ribosomal subunits. The most common of these is the gene *RPS19* which accounts for about 25% of cases. Corticosteroids are the first line of treatment. Iron chelation is required for chronically transfused

---

Box 11.4 Causes of pure red cell aplasia

Congenital
- Diamond–Blackfan syndrome (also called congenital erythroblastopenia or erythrogenesis imperfecta)

Acquired
- Idiopathic (the most common)
- Viral infections: parvovirus B19, Epstein–Barr virus, hepatitis
- Drugs and chemicals: phenytoin sodium, azathioprine, erythropoietin, benzene
- Thymoma
- Pregnancy
- Lymphoid malignancies, e.g. chronic lymphocytic leukaemia
- Other malignant diseases: carcinoma of the bronchus, breast, stomach and thyroid
- Autoimmune disorders such as systemic lupus erythematosus

patients. Allogeneic stem cell transplantation may be curative, and is normally reserved for patients with transfusion dependence.

Acquired PRCA may present as an acute self-limiting condition (for example, when it follows a parvovirus B19 infection) or as a chronic disorder. The reticulocytopenia that follows parvovirus B19 infection in normal individuals does not significantly lower the haemoglobin level because of the long half-life of red cells in the circulation. However, in patients with haemolytic anaemia, in whom red cell survival is reduced, parvovirus infection leads to severe anaemia which may be life-threatening. Patients with this complication present with severe pallor, white sclerae (normally icteric in chronic haemolysis) and other symptoms of severe anaemia.

Immunocompromised patients (e.g. due to immunosuppressive medication, HIV or post stem cell transplant) may have difficulty clearing the virus and therefore may also develop a significant drop in haemoglobin level accompanied by a marked reticulocytopenia. Such patients with persistent parvovirus B19 infection often have a good response to intravenous immunoglobulin.

Immunological mechanisms, both cellular and humoral, appear to be responsible for the majority of patients with chronic PRCA. The first-line treatment after no evidence of recovery for 4–6 weeks is corticosteroids, with or without ciclosporin. Responses have been reported to rituximab when PRCA occurs secondary to B-cell lymphoproliferative disorders. Other agents occasionally used include cyclophosphamide, ATG and the anti-CD52 directed antibody alemtuzumab. Allogeneic stem cell transplant is very occasionally used in refractory patients. For patients with a thymoma, resection is normally recommended and all patients require appropriate cross-sectional imaging to exclude this. PRCA in the context of pregnancy normally resolves on delivery.

A small number of patients with renal failure who have been given subcutaneous recombinant human erythropoietin (rhEpo) have developed red cell aplasia. This arose due to the development of neutralizing antierythropoietin antibodies when some batches of rhEpo were used. Once this was recognized and these formulations withdrawn, acquired red cell aplasia in the context of rhEpo use has become exceptionally rare.

12

Stem cell transplantation and cellular therapy

LEARNING OBJECTIVES

After reading this chapter, you should be able to:

✔ describe the use of stem cell infusion following high-dose or myeloablative chemotherapy

✔ recognize the difference between autologous and allogeneic stem cell transplant and the importance of the graft-vs-tumour effect

✔ understand the concept of CAR T-cell therapy, including its potential complications.

Haematopoietic stem cell transplantation (HSCT) is a therapeutic strategy for a variety of haematological and non-haematological disorders, which involves obliterating a patient's haematopoietic and immune system by chemotherapy, with or without radiotherapy. The marrow is then reconstituted, either with haematopoietic cells from a donor individual (a process referred to as an allogeneic stem cell transplant) or with the patient's own haematopoietic cells which have previously been harvested (autologous stem cell transplant). Cells used in HSCT may be harvested directly from the bone marrow, from the peripheral blood following stem cell mobilization, or from umbilical cord. The indications for autologous and allogeneic stem cell transplant differ, and are summarized in Table 12.1.

In recent years, another cellular therapy has become part of mainstream clinical practice in haematology: chimeric antigen receptor T (CAR T)-cell therapy. CAR T-cell therapy involves the genetic engineering of a patient's own T cells to express a synthetic receptor which targets a tumour antigen. Following expansion of the cells *in vitro*, these are then reinfused back into the patient following lymphodepleting chemotherapy. CAR T-cell therapy is now part of the standard treatment pathway for certain patients with relapsed or refractory acute lymphoblastic leukaemia and some types of non-Hodgkin lymphoma and it is likely that many more diseases will be treated in this fashion in the future.

Haematology Lecture Notes, Eleventh Edition. Deborah Hay, Andrew King and Michael Desborough.
© 2023 John Wiley & Sons Ltd. Published 2023 by John Wiley & Sons Ltd.
Companion website: www.wiley.com/go/Hay/Haematology/11e

Table 12.1 Diseases for which allogeneic and autologous bone marrow transplantation (BMT) may be considered.

Indications for BMT	Allogeneic	Autologous	Notes
Malignant			
Acute lymphoblastic leukaemia	+	–	For high-risk cases, in first remission; in second remission following relapse
Acute myeloid leukaemia	+	–	For high-risk cases, in first remission; in second remission following relapse
Chronic myeloid leukaemia	+	–	If refractory to multiple tyrosine kinase inhibitors
Myelodysplasia	+	–	If high risk and fit
Myelofibrosis	+	–	If high risk and fit
Myeloma	–	+	Autologous stem cell transplant standard of care in first remission; allogeneic stem cell transplant rarely performed in young fit patients
Hodgkin lymphoma	+	+	Autologous stem cell transplant standard of care following relapse; allogeneic stem cell transplant may be performed if refractory or relapsed following autograft
Non-Hodgkin lymphoma	+	+	Autologous stem cell transplant standard of care following relapse. Autologous stem cell transplant performed in first remission in some subtypes (e.g. PTCL, MCL). Allogeneic stem cell transplant may be performed in certain relapsed/refractory cases
Non-malignant			
Aplastic anaemia	+	–	Dependent upon age, fitness and donor availability
Thalassaemia	+	–	
Sickle cell anaemia	+	–	

MCL, mantle cell lymphoma; PTCL, peripheral T-cell lymphoma.

Collection of stem cells for HSCT

Peripheral blood stem cell collection

This is now the preferred method for collection of stem cells for both autologous and allogeneic stem cell transplant, and the majority of stem cells (70–90%) are harvested in this fashion.

Under normal circumstances, peripheral blood contains too few stem cells to allow collection of sufficient numbers for transplant and growth factor support is therefore required to enable a sufficient yield.

Patients undergoing autologous stem cell transplant often have a course of chemotherapy, and then 9–10 days of granulocyte colony stimulating factor (GCSF) treatment to stimulate a rise in the white cell count. In patients who have inadequate mobilization of stem cells (measured by CD34+ cells from the peripheral blood), plerixafor, a drug which inhibits stem cell adhesion within the stem cell niche, may also be given. Cells are collected using a cell separator machine connected to the patient, either using peripheral cannulae or via a central line (Figure 12.1).

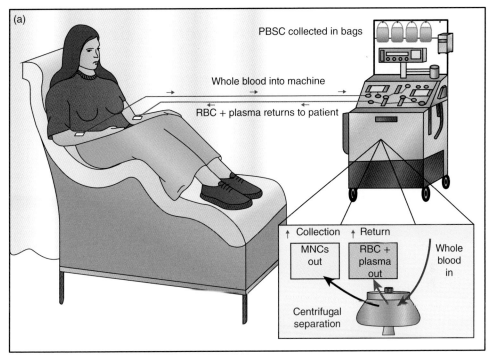

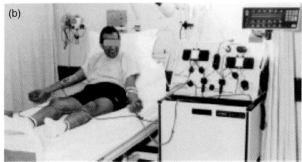

Figure 12.1 The collection of peripheral blood stem cells (PBSC) using a COBE® Spectra apheresis machine. MNC, mononuclear cell; RBC, red blood cell.

White cells are collected within the machines and red cells, platelets and plasma are returned to the patient. Collection takes around 4–5 hours and can be repeated daily for 1–3 days. Some patients fail to mobilize sufficient stem cells: this is more common in elderly patients and those who have required multiple prior lines of chemotherapy.

Donors for allogeneic stem cell transplant are given GCSF alone, normally for 4 days, and then have their stem cells collected in the same way as autologous stem cell donation. Plerixafor is not approved for use in healthy stem cell donors.

Bone marrow collection

In a few disorders (for example, aplastic anaemia), bone marrow-derived stem cells are preferred for stem cell transplantation as they lead to a slightly better outcome. Allogeneic donors who fail to mobilize sufficient stem cells peripherally may also occasionally require bone marrow collection as an emergency procedure to ensure sufficient stem cells and avoid poor or failed engraftment. Donors are also offered the choice of peripheral stem cell or bone marrow collection, with a small proportion opting for the latter.

In such circumstances, the donor is given a general anaesthetic and two operators then remove 500–1200 mL of marrow from each side of the pelvis. The marrow is anticoagulated to prevent clotting. There is typically heavy red cell contamination and the harvested product may therefore require red cell depletion, dependent upon the blood group of the donor and recipient.

Umbilical cord blood

Umbilical cords represent an important resource for patients without a sibling or unrelated donor and there are more than 150 cord blood banks, with 750 000 cord blood samples stored worldwide. Following appropriate consent, which is taken antenatally, cord blood is collected at delivery, then processed and frozen.

Autologous stem cell transplantation

The principle of autologous stem cell transplantation is to allow delivery of a high dose of chemotherapy which would otherwise be expected to lead to prolonged bone marrow aplasia. Stem cells are harvested prior to treatment and then reinfused, thereby shortening the predicted period of aplasia to approximately 14 days, during which patients can be supported with blood products and antibiotics as necessary.

Autografting continues to have a major role in the treatment of haematological malignancies, including myeloma in first remission (where it prolongs remission and improves overall survival) and in relapsed Hodgkin and non-Hodgkin lymphoma (where it may be curative following salvage chemotherapy; see Table 12.1). Transplant-related mortality is typically <5%.

Conditioning

This refers to the chemotherapy given immediately before the infusion of haematopoietic stem cells. In myeloma, the conditioning used is the alkylator melphalan given at a high dose. In lymphoma (including both Hodgkin and non-Hodgkin lymphoma), the most common conditioning used contains carmustine (BCNU), etoposide, cytarabine and melphalan, referred to by the acronym BEAM. This lasts for 7 days in total.

Allogeneic stem cell transplant

In allogeneic stem cell transplant, stem cells are harvested from another individual and then infused into the patient following conditioning chemotherapy. In malignant conditions, in addition to the antitumour effect of the conditioning chemotherapy, the lymphocytes from the graft exert an immune effect against the recipient's residual tumour cells: this 'graft-versus-leukaemia or lymphoma' (GvL) effect serves as a form of immunotherapy and explains the higher chance of cure when compared to chemotherapy alone. It can be seen, therefore, that the rationale for autologous and allogeneic transplantation strategies are very different.

An important aspect of allogeneic stem cell transplantation is balancing this therapeutic GvL effect against the adverse immune effects of the donor lymphocytes on other organ systems (referred to as graft-versus-host disease, GvHD). Allogeneic stem cell transplant is considerably more toxic than autologous stem cell transplant and transplant-related mortality is normally quoted at around 15–20%.

The HLA system and donor selection

Matching of the human leucocyte antigens (HLA) between donor and recipient permits allogeneic stem cell transplantation. The short arm of chromosome 6 (6p) contains a cluster of genes known as the major histocompatibility complex (MHC) or the HLA region. HLA proteins are divided into two types: class I and class II. Class I molecules (HLA-A, -B and -C) present antigen to CD8+ T cells and class II molecules (HLA-DR, DQ and DP) present to CD4+ T cells. Class I antigens are found on most nucleated cells; class II antigens are more restricted, being expressed on B lymphocytes, monocytes, macrophages and activated T cells.

The inheritance of the class I and class II loci is closely linked, with one set of loci inherited from each parent. Each sibling of a potential stem cell transplant recipient therefore has a one in four chance of being HLA matched. Occasionally, there may be crossing over of genes in meiosis which may lead to unexpected discrepancies.

Many patients will not have a suitable HLA-matched sibling donor and an unrelated volunteer donor is needed to provide stem cells. In 1974, the first registry for unrelated donors was established in London by Shirley Nolan, whose son, Anthony Nolan, required an allogeneic stem cell transplant for a rare inherited immunodeficiency. In the 1980s and 1990s, several countries established donor registries, and there are now over 30 million potential registered donors across the world. When searching for an unrelated donor, the aim is to match HLA-A, -B, -C, -DR and -DQ (referred to as a 10/10 match). It is also possible to transplant patients with one mismatched antigen, referred to as a 9/10 match, although this carries a higher risk of complications.

Between 70% and 80% of all patients typically have a suitable unrelated donor identified, although this is much lower in some ethnic groups, which are under-represented on the registry. In patients without an unrelated donor, it is possible to use a haploidentical related donor. In a haploidentical transplant, the donor, who is always a relative (for example, a parent, sibling or child), shares an HLA haplotype with the recipient (i.e. is a 5/10 match). Development of novel conditioning regimes has permitted the use of such donors. The most important aspect is post-transplant cyclophosphamide, which specifically targets the alloreactive donor T cells *in vivo*.

Cord blood transplants may also be used in patients without a related or unrelated HLA-matched donor. Cord blood transplants are more permissive of HLA mismatch and tend to have lower rates of graft-versus-host disease. Ideally, cord units are matched across HLA-A, -B, -C and DR (8/8) although it is possible to use cords with up to three antigens mismatched. For adult patients, two cords are normally required to ensure an adequate cell dose. Time to engraftment is usually delayed in comparison to other types of transplant, and there is consequently a higher rate of infectious complications.

Conditioning

Myeloablative conditioning regimes consist of chemotherapy (typically alkylating agents such as cyclophosphamide and busulfan), sometimes with total body irradiation (TBI, fractionated over a number of days) which irreversibly destroys the haemopoietic function of the bone marrow and is also lymphodepleting to permit engraftment of donor cells. Because of the high doses of chemotherapy and radiotherapy, the upper age limit of most myeloablative conditioning regimes is around 40–45,

although some protocols may be used in patients up to the age of 55–60.

Reduced-intensity conditioning (RIC) consists of lower doses of chemotherapy (sometimes with radiotherapy), which causes a transient aplasia and lymphodepletion but does not completely destroy the host bone marrow. The aim of these transplants is to permit donor engraftment with lower toxicity, allowing a GvL effect, which then may mediate a long-term cure. This has extended the possible age range of allogeneic transplantation for patients up to 75.

Following conditioning chemotherapy, the stem cells are infused into a vein, from which they home to the marrow and gradually engraft.

GvHD prevention

An essential component of allogeneic stem cell transplant is prevention of graft-versus-host disease. This is a consequence of the immunological attack mounted against the recipient's own tissues by donor lymphocytes. Alongside conditioning chemotherapy, the monoclonal antibody alemtuzumab (which targets CD52, a marker of mature lymphocytes) is often given, which then T cell depletes the donor cells *in vivo* after infusion. Antithymocyte globulin (ATG) is also used in a similar fashion before transplant. Post transplant, all patients receive a calcineurin inhibitor (ciclosporin or tacrolimus), providing further inhibition of lymphocyte function. Prevention of GvHD whilst maintaining the GvL effect is an active area of research, and GvHD prevention continues to evolve.

Complications

Peri-transplant

Following conditioning chemotherapy in both autologous and allogeneic stem cell transplantation, there is a temporary period of aplasia typically lasting 2–3 weeks whilst the new stem cells expand and populate the marrow. Red cells and platelet transfusions are required; these are irradiated to avoid the rare complication of transfusion-associated GvHD (see also Chapter 15). Patients are at high risk of infection which may be life-threatening. Mucositis due to the conditioning chemotherapy may be severe, and affected patients may need nutritional support.

Cytomegalovirus (CMV)

Prior to the development of routine screening for asymptomatic CMV infection and effective prophylaxis for seropositive recipients (letermovir), CMV was a major cause of morbidity and mortality in allogeneic BMT patients. Infection may be due to reactivation in a seropositive recipient, or transmission of infection from a seropositive donor. Matching of CMV serostatus is an important part of donor selection, with a mismatched donor and recipient having a higher mortality. CMV may cause hepatitis, retinitis, pneumonitis and marrow failure. Centres now routinely monitor for CMV infection weekly (normally for at least the first 12 weeks), and intervene with antiviral treatment when CMV is detected, prior to development of symptoms.

Other infections

Reactivation of herpes simplex (HSV) and varicella zoster virus (VZV) would be almost universal without adequate prophylaxis (aciclovir). Patients may occasionally develop viral strains resistant to aciclovir requiring other treatments. Reactivation of the polyomavirus BK virus may lead to haemorrhagic cystitis and renal failure. Fungal infections including *Candida* and *Aspergillus* are common without adequate prophylaxis. *Pneumocystis jirovecii* is a later cause of respiratory infection (typically after the first 30 days) and is prevented by prophylaxis with cotrimoxazole. Bacterial infections may occur at any stage, but are particularly common during the first month, and most centres use antibacterial prophylaxis (for example, ciprofloxacin) when patients are neutropenic.

Graft-vs-host disease

As described above, graft-versus-host disease is caused by donor-derived immune cells, in particular T lymphocytes, reacting against recipient tissues. Its incidence is affected by HLA mismatch, the type of GvHD prophylaxis used during conditioning and after transplant, and some other donor and recipient factors (for example, a female to male recipient has a higher rate of GvHD). There are two main syndromes: acute GvHD and chronic GvHD.

In acute GvHD, originally defined as occurring in the first 100 days after transplantation, there is a particular pattern of disease affecting the skin, gastrointestinal tract and liver. The skin rash, which is the most common manifestation, is maculopapular and affects the face, palms, soles and ears although it can affect the whole body. Diarrhoea can be severe, with the volume sometimes exceeding 3 L. In the most severe cases, there is ileus and gastrointestinal bleeding. Nausea is a common manifestation of upper GI GvHD. In acute liver GvHD, there is a cholestatic picture, with the bilirubin and alkaline phosphatase being raised to a greater extent than the transaminases. During a transplant, there is a wide differential for these symptoms (including chemotherapy effects, drugs and infection) and a biopsy is often necessary to confirm the diagnosis. Treatment is typically corticosteroids and careful supportive care; in the 50% of patients who respond poorly to steroids, there are multiple other immunosuppressive treatment options available. Severe acute GvHD remains a significant cause of morbidity and mortality post transplant. Many patients (up to 40%) may experience some acute GvHD, although severe GvHD is relatively uncommon (10–15% of patients).

In chronic GvHD, defined as occurring 100 days after transplant, the skin, GI tract and liver may also be involved although it is possible for any organ to be affected. The pattern of disease is somewhat different from that seen in acute GvHD, with skin manifestations including scleroderma changes and ulceration. The mouth (with ulceration and lichen changes), eyes (with corneal inflammation) and joints may also be severely affected. The immune system is impaired, with an increased risk of infection, often exacerbated by immunosuppressive treatment. Pulmonary complications include progressive, irreversible obstruction (bronchiolitis obliterans organising pneumonia; BOOP) which is very challenging to treat and life-limiting. Treatment for cGvHD normally includes corticosteroids first line, with other potential treatment options being similar to those used in aGvHD. Extracorporeal photopheresis in particular is often used with good effect, although treatment may need to continue for years. In severe cGvHD, the prognosis is poor and there is often a significant impact upon quality of life. The incidence is similar to acute GvHD, and patients who have had acute GvHD have a higher chance of developing chronic GvHD.

It is increasingly recognized that aside from the distinct acute and chronic GvHD syndromes, originally defined by their proximity to transplant, there may be overlap cases in which there are features of both acute and chronic GvHD in the same patient.

Sinusoidal obstruction syndrome (SOS) of the liver

Sinusoidal obstruction syndrome of the liver, previously referred to as veno-occlusive disease, manifests during the first few weeks after transplant and is characterized by jaundice, fluid retention (manifesting as weight gain and ascites) and tender hepatomegaly. It occurs following damage to hepatocytes and the sinusoidal endothelium due to conditioning chemotherapy, which then leads to blockage of the sinusoids. It is more common with certain conditioning regimens and in patients with pre-existing liver disease.

Graft failure

In a small number of patients, the donor stem cells fail to grow and repopulate the bone marrow, leaving the patient aplastic. The risk of this is increased in certain conditions (for example, aplastic anaemia and myelofibrosis). Reduced-intensity conditioning, the use of T-cell depletion (such as alemtuzumab), HLA-mismatched donors (including haploidentical transplants) and cord blood transplants also increase the risk. Graft failure is an emergency necessitating a second transplant and has a high mortality due to the risk of infection.

Post-transplant lymphoproliferative disease (PTLD)

Polyclonal or monoclonal lymphoid proliferation of the bone marrow may occur due to EBV reactivation as a consequence of the immunosuppression used during transplantation. A number of patients may develop lymphoma related to this. Transplant centres now monitor EBV viral loads routinely in order to intervene prior to the development of lymphoma. Treatment of EBV viraemia includes withdrawal of immunosuppression (if feasible) and the anti-CD20 antibody rituximab, which targets B lymphocytes (which serve as the EBV reservoir). Patients who develop lymphoma sometimes require conventional cytotoxic chemotherapy.

Late complications

The most common cause of death post allogeneic stem cell transplant in malignant disorders remains relapse of the original disease. The majority of relapses (>80%) happen in the first year after transplant. Endocrine complications including hypothyroidism, growth failure, impaired sexual development and infertility may occur; this is more common when TBI conditioning is used. Cataracts may also occur in patients who have received TBI. The risk of secondary malignancies is increased including skin, solid organ tumours and non-Hodgkin lymphoma. Secondary iron overload may occur due to repeated red cell transfusion, and patients may require venesections following red cell recovery. There is a life-time risk of increased bacterial infection, particularly when TBI is used (which typically renders patients hyposplenic) and it is recommended that oral penicillin prophylaxis is used lifelong in such patients. Patients require revaccination after transplantation, including childhood vaccinations.

Donor lymphocyte infusions (DLI)

Following allogeneic stem cell transplant, the recipient's blood may show the presence of both donor and recipient cells (referred to as chimerism). It is possible using DNA analysis of short-tandem repeats (which differ between individuals) to estimate the degree of chimerism, which is conventionally expressed as a percentage, with 100% meaning that only donor cells are present. It is now well established that there is an increased risk of relapse when there is mixed T-cell chimerism (as there is then a suboptimal GvL effect) following withdrawal of immunosuppression. In such situations, lymphocyte infusions from the original allograft donor may be given directly to the patient in escalating doses every 3 months, in an attempt to convert the patient to full donor T-cell chimerism. Administration of the lymphocyte infusion itself is usually trivial and done as a day case, although there is a risk of both acute and chronic GvHD developing in the following 6–12 weeks, which may be severe.

Because donor lymphocytes mediate the GvL affect, they are also used in relapsed disease or situations where there is rising measurable residual disease (Figure 12.2). There is a large difference in the outcome of different diseases treated by DLI, with chronic myeloid leukaemia (CML) being the most sensitive and acute lymphoblastic leukaemia rarely

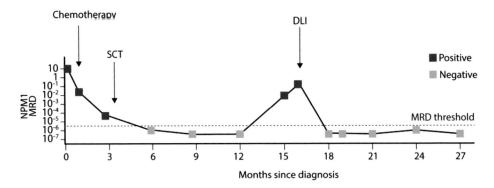

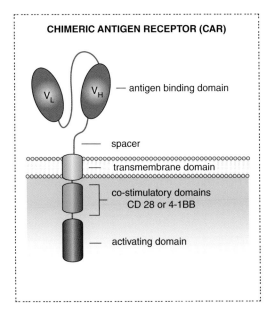

Figure 12.2 Monitoring of measurable residual disease in NPM1 mutated AML. After induction chemotherapy and an allogeneic stem cell transplant, the patient was MRD negative. Following rising NPM1 transcript levels, administration of a donor lymphocyte infusion returned the patient to an MRD negative remission, illustrating the GvL effect. DLI, donor lymphocyte infusion; MRD, minimal residual disease; SCT, stem cell transplantation.

responding. Donor lymphocytes may sometimes lead to a long-term cure, although are best administered when there are low levels of disease, rather than frank relapse.

Chimeric antigen receptor T-cell therapy

An emerging therapeutic field within haematology is the engineering of autologous T cells to express receptors which target antigens on malignant cells. Following lymphodepleting chemotherapy, these modified cells are then reinfused into patients where they rapidly expand, often eliciting potent anti-tumour activity. The ideal target antigen is selectively expressed only on tumour cells to avoid off-target side-effects. Currently, the majority of CAR T cells in routine use target the B-cell antigen CD19 and are used to treat B-acute lymphoblastic leukaemia (B-ALL), diffuse large B-cell lymphoma and mantle cell lymphoma. Broadly, about 40–50% of patients with multiply relapsed/refractory disease can be cured with this approach. Other products in development or recently approved target myeloma-specific antigens or antigens on acute myeloid leukaemia. CAR T cells designed to target multiple antigens (e.g. both CD19 and CD22 in B-ALL) may be useful in the setting of malignancies where cell populations lacking a single antigen become dominant in response to treatment. It is likely that the number of CAR T products and indications will increase over the next decade.

Figure 12.3 A chimeric antigen receptor construct, The antigen-binding domain consists of a variable heavy (V_H) and variable light chain (V_L) region.
Source: Courtesy of Dr Caroline Watson.

CAR T cells are artificial constructs which comprise an antigen recognition ectodomain (a single-chain variable immunoglobulin fragment) and an activation endodomain, linked by a spacer and a transmembrane domain (Figure 12.3).

Second-generation products (which are the only products in clinical use) also incorporate a costimulatory endodomain.

Administration of CAR T-cell therapy

Production of CAR T cells involves cell collection by leucapheresis (using the same method as for stem cell collection), followed by removal of myeloid cells, T-cell enrichment and activation, transgene incorporation into the T cells to produce the CAR construct, and *ex vivo* expansion (Figure 12.4). The manufacture of the cells, normally undertaken commercially, takes 4–6 weeks and patients will often need bridging chemotherapy or radiotherapy in this period. Following successful manufacture of cells, patients are given low-dose conditioning chemotherapy, causing lymphodepletion to allow CAR T-cell expansion *in vivo* following cell infusion. Following CAR T-cell infusion, patients are monitored for complications.

Complications

CAR T-cell therapy has two specific acute and potentially life-threatening toxicities: cytokine release syndrome (CRS) and immune effector cell-associated neurotoxicity syndrome (ICANS).

Cytokine release syndrome

Cytokine release syndrome is a systemic reaction, caused by the activation and expansion of CAR T cells, the lysis of tumour cells and the activation of other immune cells including monocytes and macrophages with florid cytokine release. The majority of patients will experience CRS to some degree; although it can occur up to 3 weeks following CAR T infusion, the typical onset is within the first 48–72 hours. Clinically, patients often develop a flu-like syndrome with fever (often >40°C), fatigue, headache and arthralgia. In more severe cases, there is haemodynamic instability with hypotension, capillary leak leading to hypoxia, and organ dysfunction.

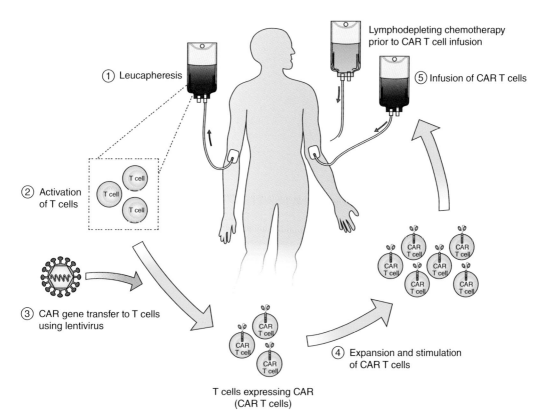

Figure 12.4 Manufacture of CAR T cells. The entire process from leucapheresis to cell infusion can take up to 6 weeks.
Source: Courtesy of Dr Caroline Watson.

Mild cases may be managed with antipyretics, empiric antibiotics and fluid boluses. More severe cases, characterized by refractory hypotension and worsening hypoxia, require treatment with the IL-6 antagonist tocilizumab which has a high response rate. Failure to respond to tocilizumab within 24–36 hours necessitates high-dose steroids. At least 20% of patients develop severe CRS requiring treatment in an intensive care environment, and some patients require multiorgan support including intubation and ventilation. Close liaison with intensive care is important, as patients may deteriorate rapidly.

Immune effector cell-associated neurotoxicity syndrome

In this syndrome, it is thought that increased permeability of the blood–brain barrier due to inflammation allows high concentrations of inflammatory cytokines into the cerebrospinal fluid (CSF). CAR T-cells are also found in the CSF during episodes, and may play a direct role. Patients manifest impaired attention, language disturbance, confusion and disorientation. Headache, tremors and agitation are also seen. In severe cases, seizures, motor weakness, increased intracranial pressure and cerebral oedema leading to coma occur. Up to 60% of patients may be affected depending upon the product used, usually in the 4–7 days after CAR T infusion.

Patients are managed in conjunction with neurologists. Cranial imaging, CSF examination and electroencephalogram (EEG) form part of the routine work-up, mainly to exclude other causes of neurotoxicity.

Prophylactic antiepileptics are started in all patients. For more severe cases, corticosteroids (typically dexamethasone) are administered. ICU monitoring may be necessary.

Other complications

Sometimes patients react to the infusion of cells, although profound allergic reactions are unusual. Tumour lysis syndrome is possible in patients with a high tumour burden. When CD19 CAR T cells are used, prolonged B-cell aplasia is very common, and is a marker of CAR T-cell persistence. Patients may require intravenous immunoglobulin replacement therapy if they suffer recurrent bacterial infections, although in practice this is rare. Severe pancytopenia (for a longer duration than expected due to the lymphodepleting chemotherapy) is extremely common and can last several weeks after CAR T-cell infusion. The mechanism underlying this remains uncertain. Prolonged cytopenias are managed with growth factors and supportive medications including antifungal prophylaxis.

Future directions

A mechanism of CAR T-cell failure currently is loss of the CD19 antigen or epitope despite adequate persistence of transferred cells. Administering CAR T cells against multiple targets (for example, both CD19 and CD22 in B-ALL) may circumvent this problem, and is currently in late-phase clinical trials.

13

Haemostasis and bleeding disorders

LEARNING OBJECTIVES

After reading this chapter, you should be able to:

✔ describe the function of platelets and the relationship between the platelet count in the peripheral blood and the likelihood of abnormal bleeding

✔ recognize the diseases associated with thrombocytopenia and platelet function disorders

✔ describe the main sequence of events in the coagulation pathways

✔ understand normal fibrinolysis and the principles of fibrinolytic therapy

✔ describe the principles underlying the prothrombin time and activated partial thromboplastin time

✔ outline the principles of investigation of a patient suspected of having a haemostatic defect

✔ describe the mode of inheritance, clinical presentation, method of diagnosis and principles of treatment of haemophilia A (factor VIII deficiency), haemophilia B (factor IX deficiency) and von Willebrand disease

✔ understand the effects of vitamin K deficiency and liver disease on the clotting mechanisms

✔ describe the alterations in the haemostatic and fibrinolytic mechanisms associated with disseminated intravascular coagulation and its causes.

Normal haemostasis

The cessation of bleeding following trauma to blood vessels results from three processes.

- The contraction of vessel walls.
- The formation of a platelet plug at the site of the break in the vessel wall.
- The formation of a fibrin clot.

The clot forms within and around the platelet aggregates and results in a firm haemostatic plug. The relative importance of these three processes probably varies according to the size of the vessels involved. Thus, in bleeding from a minor wound, the formation of a haemostatic plug is probably sufficient in itself, whereas in larger vessels, contraction of the vessel walls also plays a part in haemostasis. The initial plug is formed almost entirely of platelets, but this is friable and is subsequently stabilized by fibrin formation.

Haematology Lecture Notes, Eleventh Edition. Deborah Hay, Andrew King and Michael Desborough.
© 2023 John Wiley & Sons Ltd. Published 2023 by John Wiley & Sons Ltd.
Companion website: www.wiley.com/go/Hay/Haematology/11e

Classlfication of haemostatic defects

The action of platelets and the clotting mechanism are closely intertwined in the prevention of bleeding. However, it can be helpful to consider abnormalities in haemostasis resulting in bleeding as arising from defects in one of three processes.

- Thrombocytopenia (a low platelet count) – the most common cause.
- Abnormal platelet function.
- A defect in the clotting factors – the second most common cause.

For the rest of this chapter, we will discuss first the normal process of primary haemostasis, i.e. the formation of the platelet plug and its disorders, and then move on to the mechanisms and diseases of fibrin clot formation, also termed secondary or definitive haemostasis.

Formation of the platelet plug – the process of primary haemostasis

The main function of platelets is to form a haemostatic plug at sites of damage to vascular endothelium (Figure 13.1). Platelet production in the bone marrow is stimulated by thrombopoietin, a hormone secreted by the liver. Thrombopoietin stimulates megakaryocyte proliferation and differentiation into platelets (see also Chapter 1). When released into the blood, platelets have an average life of 7–10 days before they are either consumed as part of the formation of a platelet plug or removed from the circulation by splenic macrophages.

There are three stages to the formation of the platelet plug. The first is platelet adhesion in which, following injury to a blood vessel, collagen and von Willebrand factor, a glycoprotein synthesized in the endothelial cells and essential for normal haemostasis, are exposed. Von Willebrand factor attaches to a

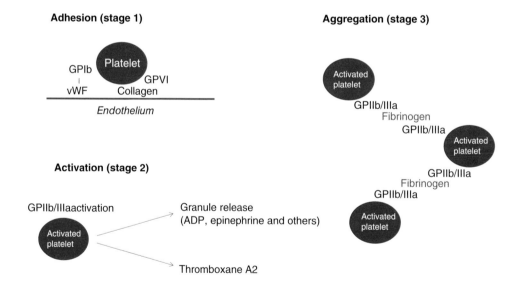

Figure 13.1 Formation of a platelet plug. The first stage is platelet adhesion. Initially, endothelial von Willebrand factor (vWF) binds to platelet glycoprotein (GP) 1b, tethering the platelet. The platelet binds to subendothelial collagen through its glycoprotein VI receptor. The second stage is activation when platelets activate their glycoprotein IIb/IIIa receptors and release granules and thromboxane. These activate other nearby platelets. The third stage is platelet aggregation when activated platelets bind together through their glycoprotein IIb/IIIa receptors (and via fibrinogen) to form a platelet plug. ADP, adenosine diphosphate.

specific glycoprotein on the surface of platelets, platelet factor 1b, tethering the platelet to the site of endothelial injury (see Figure 13.1). Platelets then also bind to collagen directly through glycoprotein VI receptors on their surface.

The second stage is platelet activation when the platelets release the prothrombotic contents of their intracellular granules along with thromboxane – a powerful thrombotic mediator which activates platelets and causes vasoconstriction. The third stage is platelet aggregation when platelets bind together via fibrinogen through their glycoprotein IIb/IIIa receptors.

Defects in primary haemostasis

While the processes of primary and secondary haemostasis are closely intertwined, there is some justification for considering them separately in order to understand the ways in which haemostasis can be deranged in disease states. Dysfunction of primary haemostasis typically gives a pattern of bleeding which is mucosal, for example causing epistaxis, gastrointestinal bleeding or menorrhagia. Bleeding within the skin, causing purpura or petechiae, is also common.

Thrombocytopenic and non-thrombocytopenic purpura

'Purpura' is the collective term for bleeding into the skin or mucous membranes. Patients with purpura can be separated into those with low platelet counts (thrombocytopenic) and those with normal platelet counts (non-thrombocytopenic). The non-thrombocytopenic group can be subdivided into those patients who have qualitative platelet defects (including von Willebrand disease) and a group who have vascular abnormalities. The latter is a miscellaneous group and contains congenital disorders such as hereditary haemorrhagic telangiectasia (Figure 13.2) and the Ehlers–Danlos syndrome, acquired diseases such as Henoch–Schönlein purpura (a vasculitis) and scurvy.

Causes of thrombocytopenia

The mechanisms leading to thrombocytopenia are:

- a failure of platelet production by bone marrow megakaryocytes
- a shortened lifespan of the platelets
- increased pooling of platelets in an enlarged spleen.

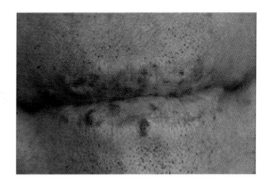

Figure 13.2 Vascular malformations (reddish purple) on the lips of a patient with hereditary haemorrhagic telangiectasia; such lesions are found throughout the body and increase in number with advancing age. This rare condition is inherited as an autosomal dominant characteristic and may lead to recurrent gastrointestinal haemorrhage and chronic iron deficiency anaemia.

The distinction between the first two of these possibilities can be made by assessing the number of megakaryocytes in a marrow aspirate or trephine biopsy of the marrow. The causes of thrombocytopenia are given in Box 13.1.

Failure of platelet production

If megakaryocytes are few or absent, it may be assumed that platelet production is at fault. The bone marrow smears may also reveal other features that indicate the nature of the disease if evidence has not already been obtained from the peripheral blood. Thus, there may be a generalized aplasia of the bone marrow (aplastic anaemia) or a selective decrease in megakaryocytes caused by certain drugs (e.g. chlorothiazides, tolbutamide), alcohol excess and certain viruses (e.g. Epstein–Barr virus, measles, varicella, cytomegalovirus). Another cause of reduced platelet production is marked infiltration of the marrow by malignant cells or fibrous tissue. Reduced platelet production may also occur in patients with normal or increased numbers of megakaryocytes when there is ineffective megakaryopoiesis, as in severe vitamin B12 or folate deficiency or in myelodysplastic syndromes.

Shortened platelet survival

If the megakaryocytes in the marrow are numerous, then the thrombocytopenia is usually caused by an excessive rate of removal of platelets from the

> **Box 13.1 Causes of thrombocytopenia**
>
> *Failure of platelet production*
> - Aplastic anaemia
> - Drugs
> - Viruses
> - Defective maturation of the myeloid component of the marrow (e.g. myelodysplasia)
> - Bone marrow infiltration (haematological and non-haematological malignancies, marrow fibrosis, storage diseases including Gaucher disease, osteopetrosis)
> - Megaloblastic anaemia from B12 or folate deficiency
> - Paroxysmal nocturnal haemoglobinuria
> - Rare hereditary thrombocytopenia syndromes (e.g. thrombocytopenia with absent radii, grey platelet syndrome, Bernard–Soulier syndrome, Wiskott–Aldrich syndrome)
>
> *Shortened platelet survival*
>
> Immune
> - Immune thrombocytopenia (ITP)
> - Secondary autoimmune thrombocytopenic purpura (systemic lupus erythematosus and other collagen diseases, lymphoproliferative diseases, HIV infection)
> - Drugs
> - Post-transfusion purpura
> - Thrombotic thrombocytopenic purpura
> - Neonatal alloimmune thrombocytopenia
>
> Non-immune
> - Disseminated intravascular coagulation
> - Increased splenic pooling

peripheral circulation. In most cases, the destruction results from autoantibodies attached to the platelet surface and the disease is termed (auto) immune thrombocytopenia (ITP). Occasionally, it is a result of intravascular platelet consumption because of disseminated intravascular coagulation (DIC) or microangiopathic haemolytic anaemia (e.g. thrombotic thrombocytopenic purpura [TTP] or the haemolytic uraemic syndrome). These conditions are considered in further detail below.

Immune thrombocytopenia

In ITP, immune-mediated destruction of platelets leads to thrombocytopenia. ITP is characterized by petechiae (Figure 13.3), bruising, spontaneous bleeding from mucous membranes and a reduction in the platelet count (without neutropenia or, usually, anaemia). The pathogenic mechanism was previously thought to be due to IgG autoantibodies that result in a shortened platelet lifespan because of premature destruction in the spleen. It is now accepted that there are more complex mechanisms, in which both impaired platelet production and T-cell-mediated effects have a role.

In children, ITP is usually seen before the age of 10 years. Two-thirds give a history of a common childhood viral infection (e.g. upper respiratory tract infection, chickenpox, measles) 2–3 weeks preceding the purpura. Platelet counts are often less than 20×10^9/L. It is diagnosed by identifying a low platelet count, with no other explanation for the thrombocytopenia and no other abnormalities on the full blood count or blood film. For children with ITP, no treatment is usually necessary. The risk of serious bleeding for children with ITP is low and the majority will spontaneously recover without treatment.

For adults, ITP is diagnosed in a similar way as for children by identifying thrombocytopenia with an otherwise normal full blood count and an otherwise normal blood film (Figure 13.4). However, a range of other diagnoses should be excluded, including HIV, hepatitis B, hepatitis C, vitamin B12 deficiency, folate deficiency, hypogammaglobulinaemia, other autoimmune disorders such as systemic lupus erythematosus and drug-induced thrombocytopenia. ITP in adults is therefore a diagnosis of exclusion. Failure to respond to ITP treatments should trigger re-evaluation of whether the diagnosis is correct. Bone marrow aspirate and trephine is not routinely performed for initial investigation of ITP, but classically, the findings

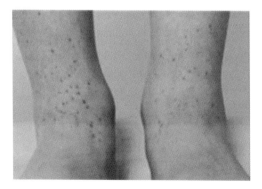

Figure 13.3 Multiple pinpoint haemorrhages (petechiae) on the legs of a patient with immune thrombocytopenic purpura (ITP).

Figure 13.4 Typical blood film
from a patient with ITP. Only one
platelet is seen and, as is often
the case in consumptive causes
of thrombocytopenia, this is
larger than normal. The red cells
and leucocytes appear normal.
MGG stain.

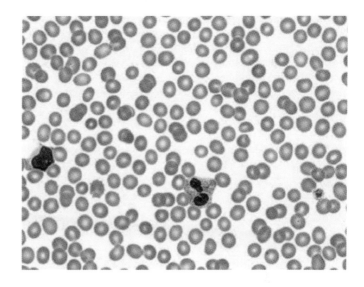

Figure 13.4 Typical blood film from a patient with ITP. Only one platelet is seen and, as is often the case in consumptive causes of thrombocytopenia, this is larger than normal. The red cells and leucocytes appear normal. MGG stain.

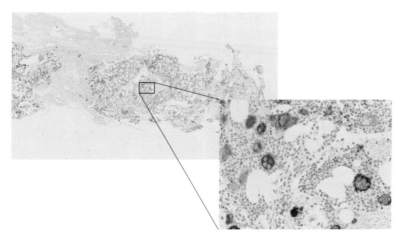

Figure 13.5 Typical bone marrow from a patient with ITP, both low- and high-power views. The marrow has been immunostained with antibody against CD61, a megakaryocyte marker, and shows a striking increase in megakaryocyte numbers.

in the bone marrow in ITP will be of increased mega-karyocyte numbers, as the bone marrow attempts to compensate for the increased destruction of platelets by producing more (Figure 13.5).

In months 0–3 after diagnosis, ITP is considered to be acute. For adults with acute ITP, there is a greater risk of major bleeding than for children, particularly when the platelet count falls below 10×10^9/L, although bleeding will sometimes occur when the platelet count is 30–50 $\times 10^9$/L. Initial treatment of acute ITP is usually with immunosuppression with corticosteroids, sometimes in combination with other agents such as mycophenolate. Where avoiding

immunosuppresion is important, it is possible to use thrombopoietin mimetics (such as romiplostim, eltrombopag and avatrombopag) as initial treatment. Approximately two-thirds of patients treated with corticosteroids will reach remission but only a minor-ity (10–20%) will have a long-term remission and relapses are common. Relapses can be treated with repeated courses of corticosteroids or other immuno-suppressant drugs.

Immune thrombocytopenic purpura that is still present in months 4–12 is known as persistent ITP and other immunosuppressant strategies are often used. When ITP lasts for more than 1 year, this is known as chronic ITP. Thrombopoietin mimetics are often considered in these circumstances. These drugs mimic the effects of thrombopoietin and stimulate the bone marrow to produce more platelets to compensate for the thrombocytopenia. In refractory cases, another option is surgical removal of the spleen to slow platelet removal from the circulation. This is effective in the majority of cases but is associated with thrombosis and life-long risks of infection so is usually only considered when medical therapy has failed.

Secondary autoimmune thrombocytopenic purpura

An autoimmune thrombocytopenia may precede other manifestations of SLE by several years and may complicate the course of SLE, other autoimmune disorders and disorders such as B-cell lymphoproliferative diseases where immune dysregulation can be seen. Patients infected with the human immunodeficiency virus (HIV) may develop either autoimmune thrombocytopenia or immune thrombocytopenia (caused by immune complexes) long before developing other characteristic features.

Drug-induced immune thrombocytopenia

Certain drugs such as heparin, gold salts, quinine, quinidine, sulfonamides or penicillins can cause a shortening of platelet lifespan in a small proportion of recipients by an immunological mechanism. Heparin-induced thrombocytopenia (HIT) is particularly important. Antibodies form against the heparin–platelet factor 4 (PF4) complex and then bind to the platelet FcγR, causing platelet activation, thrombocytopenia and an often seemingly paradoxical thrombosis (see Chapter 14).

Other immune thrombocytopenias

In the rare condition known as post-transfusion purpura, severe thrombocytopenia develops 5–8 days after a blood component transfusion as a result of the destruction of the recipient's own platelets. In this disorder, platelet-specific alloantibodies are present in the serum (most often antibodies against human platelet antigen 1a), but the explanation for the destruction of the patient's own platelets remains unclear.

Transient but potentially serious neonatal alloimmune thrombocytopenia may occur in babies of healthy mothers. The mother forms IgG alloantibodies against a fetal platelet-specific antigen (most commonly human platelet antigen 1a) which is lacking on the mother's platelets and inherited from the father; these antibodies cross the placenta and damage fetal platelets (analogous to haemolytic disease of the newborn, see Chapter 15). This condition may lead to intracerebral bleeding and, unlike haemolytic disease of the newborn, often affects a first pregnancy.

Thrombotic thrombocytopenic purpura

This rare but potentially fatal disorder is also characterized by thrombocytopenia, though with a more complex underlying mechanism involving von Willebrand factor (vWF). vWF is essential for normal platelet adhesion, as described above, and is secreted by the endothelial Weibel-Palade bodies in long multimers (amongst the largest proteins in the human body). In healthy individuals, a vWF-cleaving protease (ADAMTS13) cleaves the Tyr 842-Met 843 peptide bond in vWF to produce shorter vWF multimers. The shorter multimers are less haemostatically active.

In thrombotic thrombocytopenic purpura (TTP), an autoantibody neutralizes ADAMTS13 (or less commonly a person is born with a genetic defect in their ADAMTS13 gene) and this leads to reduction in ADAMTS13 levels. Ultra-large vWF multimers are no longer cleaved and lead to spontaneous platelet aggregation throughout the circulation. In advanced TTP, cardiac, neurological and renal damage, caused by platelet- and vWF-rich microthrombi, are often seen. Red cell trauma is also induced by a combination of endothelial activation and shear stress damage caused by the vWF microthrombi, giving a microangiopathic haemolytic anaemia.

It is essential that this condition is recognized early, because it is treatable and the untreated death rate is 90–100%. Any patients with thrombocytopenia and a microangiopathic anaemia (haemolysis with red cell fragments on the blood film) should be considered to have TTP until proven otherwise and should have urgent empirical treatment. The confirmatory test is demonstration of severely deficient ADAMTS13 activity. TTP is treated as an emergency with a combination of plasma exchange, high-dose corticosteroids and rituximab (an anti-CD20 antibody that depletes B cells, thereby addressing the underlying immune aetiology). Additionally, patients will also be considered for treatment with caplacizumab, a drug that inhibits binding between vWF and platelet glycoprotein 1b. Patients with previous TTP are followed up life-long to detect any early signs of relapse.

Other causes of thrombocytopenia and microangiopathic haemolytic anaemia include DIC (although in this condition the coagulation profile would be expected to be abnormal, see below), haemolytic uraemic syndrome, antiphospholipid syndrome, advanced liver disease and pregnancy-related microangiopathies.

Increased splenic pooling

A normal spleen contains within its microcirculation about 30% of all the blood platelets; the platelets in the splenic pool exchange freely with those in the general circulation. The splenic platelet pool increases with increasing spleen size, so that in patients with moderate to massive splenomegaly, it may hold 50–90% of all blood platelets, thus causing thrombocytopenia. Another factor contributing to the thrombocytopenia in patients with splenomegaly is an increase in plasma volume.

Abnormalities of platelet function or of von Willebrand factor

Not all patients with defects in primary haemostasis will have a low platelet count. In many cases, dysfunction of platelets or of their interaction with vWF is responsible.

Acquired defects of platelet function

Perhaps the most common defect in platelet function is that seen after ingestion of aspirin and other antiplatelet drugs. Aspirin acts by irreversibly acetylating cyclo-oxygenase and this inhibits thromboxane A2 synthesis, with a subsequent reduction in platelet aggregation. The effect of a single dose of aspirin can be detected for a week (i.e. until most of the platelets present at the time of taking the aspirin have been replaced by newly formed platelets). Clopidogrel acts

by irreversibly blocking the ADP receptor ($P2Y_{12}$) on the platelet cell membrane, which is needed for platelet aggregation. Other causes of an acquired abnormality of platelet function include chronic myeloproliferative disorders, myelodysplastic syndromes, paraproteinaemias (e.g. myeloma or Waldenström macroglobulinaemia) and uraemia.

Inherited defects of platelet function

Primary platelet function disorders are rare, and may arise as a consequence of problems with platelet membrane receptors or platelet granules. They are summarized in Table 13.1.

Von Willebrand disease

This is the most common inherited bleeding disorder. Approximately 1% of the United Kingdom population have low vWF levels, although the number with von Willebrand disease (vWF antigen or activity less than 0.30 IU/mL) and clinically relevant bleeding symptoms is closer to 1 in 10000. Most mild cases are undiagnosed. It is an autosomal disorder characterized by mild, moderate or severe bleeding. The bleeding results from either a qualitative abnormality or a deficiency of vWF. This protein has a dual function: first, it is an adhesive molecule that binds platelets to subendothelial tissues; second, it acts as a carrier for factor VIII. The reduction in vWF results in a reduction in factor VIII concentration (usually measured as clotting activity), which may be as low as 5–30% of normal, similar to that found in mild haemophilia. However, the excessive bleeding in the disease is mainly a result of the failure of the platelets to adhere rather than the concomitant factor VIII deficiency, hence its inclusion here as a disorder related principally to primary haemostasis.

Table 13.1 Inherited platelet defects.

Disorder	Pathological basis	Clinical features
Glanzmann disease	Lack of glycoprotein (GP) IIb/IIIa receptors	Autosomal recessive Normal platelet count and appearance
Bernard–Soulier disease	Lack of GP Ib receptors	Autosomal recessive. Platelets are larger than normal and usually the platelet count is reduced
May–Hegglin anomaly	Defective megakaryocyte maturation/fragmentation	Autosomal dominant; large platelets and characteristic white cell inclusions
Storage pool diseases	Various – defective platelet granule production	Mode of inheritance and clinical pattern vary according to type

The gene for vWF is on chromosome 12 and analysis of the gene has shown that there is considerable heterogeneity in the genetic defects found in vWD. Some defects result in a reduction in the plasma concentration of structurally normal vWF molecules, but others cause different qualitative abnormalities in the vWF molecule. vWD has therefore been divided into three types. In type 1 (most frequent), there is a partial reduction in vWF. In type 2, there is a functional defect in vWF. In type 3 (the rarest and most severe form of vWD) there is nearly complete absence of vWF.

Most patients have type 1 vWD, inherited as an autosomal dominant trait with variable penetrance, and are mildly affected. Spontaneous bleeding is usually confined to mucous membranes and skin and takes the form of epistaxis and ecchymoses, bleeding after dental extraction and menorrhagia. Severe haemorrhage may occur following surgical procedures. Bleeding into joints and muscles is rare except in type 3 disease, where the reduction in factor VIII half-life means this clinically resembles haemophilia A (see below).

For mildly or moderately affected patients with type 1 (and some types of type 2) disease, a vasopressin analogue desmopressin (1-deamino-8-D-arginine vasopressin, DDAVP), which stimulates a temporary increase in factor VIII and vWF by inducing the release of these factors from Weibel-Palade bodies in endothelial cells, can be used. Some patients, however, will require direct supplementation with vWF, and this may be plasma derived or recombinant. The antifibrinolytic drug tranexamic acid may be used for treating epistaxis or menorrhagia and in combination with DDAVP or vWF-containing concentrates to manage dental extractions.

Assessing primary haemostasis in patients

When seeing a patient with clinical features suggesting a defect in primary haemostasis, a good clinical history and examination are essential.

1 When did the bleeding symptoms start? This will help differentiate inherited bleeding disorders, which would be expected to start from a young age, from acquired bleeding disorders that may start later in life or only following significant haemostatic challenge. An extended family history or any history of consanguinity is important.

2 What is the patient's history of bleeding symptoms? It is helpful to enquire about nose bleeds, bleeding following minor cuts, oral bleeding, unexplained bruising, haematuria, gastrointestinal bleeding, intramuscular bleeding, intra-articular bleeding and intracranial bleeding. For women, enquire about heavy menstrual bleeding and postpartum haemorrhage. It is helpful to know if patients have ever had a tooth extraction or undergone surgery, or faced any other haemostatic challenge. Bleeding disorders related to thrombocytopenia, platelet dysfunction or von Willebrand disease typically manifest with mucocutaneous bleeding whereas clotting factor disorders such as haemophilia A often present with delayed bleeding into muscles or joints. Petechiae, which are non-blanching red marks on the skin, less than 1 mm in diameter (see Figure 13.3), are usually associated with thrombocytopenia.

3 Does the patient have any medical conditions that may be linked to bleeding, for instance liver disease or renal disease? Are they taking any medications which might affect clotting function?

After this, laboratory tests of haemostatic function are needed. Those especially useful for primary haemostasis include full blood count, blood film, platelet function analyser and von Willebrand assays.

An assessment of the number of platelets will be possible with a routine full blood count. A blood film will also enable assessment of platelet size and granularity, important for some inherited platelet disorders. The 'immature platelet fraction' is also provided by some analysers, and gives a sense of the rate of release of young platelets into the circulation – a higher number suggesting a likely consumptive explanation for any thrombocytopenia rather than a failure of production.

Historically, the effectiveness of primary haemostasis was assessed using the bleeding time – measuring the time taken for bleeding from a small superficial incision in the skin to stop bleeding. This test, rather poorly reproducible and subject to many variables, is now generally replaced by *in vitro* estimation of primary haemostasis using the platelet function analyser (PFA). In this instrument, platelets are passed through holes in a membrane coated with collagen and either adenosine diphosphate (ADP) or epinephrine, and the time taken for flow to cease is measured. The PFA closure time may be prolonged by various defects in primary haemostasis (including vWD, thrombocytopenia, anaemia and platelet function defects).

Some laboratories use the PFA to rule out a platelet defect when the pretest probability is low, but it can be normal in some platelet disorders and platelet aggregation studies are required if a platelet defect is a likely possibility, even if PFA closure times are normal. Aggregation studies assess the response of platelet-rich plasma to agonists like ADP, epinephrine, arachidonic acid, collagen and ristocetin. When the platelets in a sample aggregate in response to these agonists, more light is able to pass through the sample and this can be measured to give an estimate of response, hence the term light transmission aggregometry.

For von Willebrand disease, vWF levels can be measured directly, and its function tested by specialist clotting laboratories.

Secondary/definitive haemostasis: clotting and the coagulation cascade

Following the formation of the platelet plug, the next step in normal haemostasis is the formation of a fibrin clot within and around the platelet plug. Anionic phospholipids exposed on the surface of activated platelets enhance the speed of coagulation on the platelet surface. The clotting cascade consists of inactive zymogens that when activated become proteolytic enzymes. The cascade means that an initial small stimulus is amplified, leading to a much larger end effect.

The zymogens are denoted by a Roman numeral and the proteolytic enzymes (activated clotting factors) are denoted by a Roman numeral followed by the letter 'a'. For instance, as it becomes activated, the factor VIII zymogen becomes factor VIIIa (a proteolytic enzyme).

The clotting factors were given Roman numerals in the order they were discovered – not consistently in an order which is relevant for an understanding of their function. Moreover, some factors have been renamed when their identity and role became better understood so 'factor III' is now known as tissue factor, 'factor IV' has been shown to be calcium and 'factor VI' is in fact activated factor Va. This leaves 10 procoagulant factors of the clotting cascade: factors I (fibrinogen), II (prothrombin), V, VII, VIII, IX, X, XI, XII and XIII (Figure 13.6).

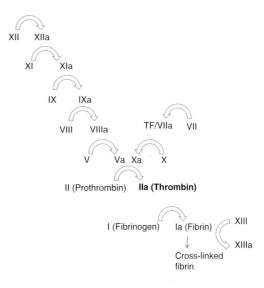

Figure 13.6 Coagulation cascade. The clotting factor zymogens are represented by Roman numerals and proteolytic enzymes (activated clotting factors) by a Roman numeral followed by the letter 'a'. TF, tissue factor.

Prothrombin time and activated partial thromboplastin time

The normal physiological processes of haemostasis are only imperfectly represented by the coagulation cascade shown in Figure 13.6; moreover, efforts to recapitulate these normal processes in the diagnostic haematology laboratory do not always accurately represent normal haemostasis. Figure 13.7 shows a simplified coagulation cascade which summarizes a process more representative of our current physiological understanding of haemostasis. Here, endothelial damage leads to exposure of tissue factor and this, in combination with factor VIIa, stimulates the formation of thrombin (factor IIa) from prothrombin (factor II) with the help of cofactors (II and X). The formation of this small amount of thrombin creates a feedback loop, whereby factors XI, IX and VIII induce the formation of a much larger burst of thrombin with the help of factors V and X. This leads to cleavage of fibrinogen (factor I), converting it to insoluble fibrin (factor Ia), the substance of which a fibrin clot is formed. Factor XIII, activated by thrombin, cross-links the fibrin strands to form a more stable clot.

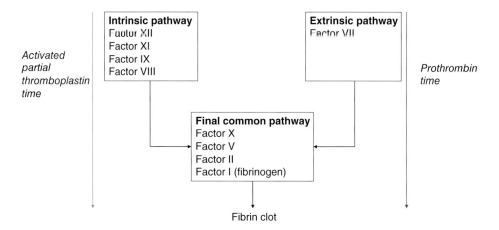

Activated partial thromboplastin time

Intrinsic pathway
Factor XII
Factor XI
Factor IX
Factor VIII

Extrinsic pathway
Factor VII

Prothrombin time

Final common pathway
Factor X
Factor V
Factor II
Factor I (fibrinogen)

Fibrin clot

Figure 13.7 Simplified coagulation cascade. The prothrombin time is the time from triggering the extrinsic pathway to forming a fibrin clot. It will be prolonged if any of the factors in the extrinsic pathway or final common pathway are deficient (or in the presence of an inhibitor such as a lupus anticoagulant). The activated partial thromboplastin time is the time from triggering the intrinsic pathway to forming a fibrin clot. It will be prolonged if any of the factors in the extrinsic pathway or final common pathway are deficient (or in the presence of an inhibitor).

The procoagulant factors of the clotting cascade can be organized into three pathways: the extrinsic pathway (also known as the tissue factor pathway), the intrinsic pathway (also known as the contact pathway) and the final common pathway (see Figure 13.7).

The extrinsic pathway only contains factor VII. The intrinsic pathway contains factors VIII, IX, XI and XII (and contact factors which may be considered redundant in normal haemostasis: prekallikrein and high molecular weight kininogen). The final common pathway contains factors I, II, V and X. Factor XIII is outside the main clotting cascade as it takes effect after the formation of fibrin.

Assessing the process of coagulation in the laboratory attempts to recapitulate this process, but is necessarily an imperfect representation of *in vivo* haemostasis. The tests used are the prothrombin time, a representation of the extrinsic or tissue factor pathway, and the activated partial thromboplastin time, which attempts to represent the intrinsic pathway.

The prothrombin time is measured by stimulating factor VII through the addition of a recombinant form of tissue factor to a sample of patient plasma. The factor VIIa which is formed triggers the factors of the final common pathway, leading to the formation of a fibrin clot. The time taken from the initial stimulation of the extrinsic pathway to the formation of the fibrin clot is the prothrombin time or PT, and deficiency of factor VII or of any factor of the final common pathway (I, II, V and X) will lead to prolongation of the prothrombin time.

The activated partial thromboplastin time is measured by stimulating factor XII through the addition of a partial thromboplastin (a phospholipid and silica, without tissue factor), which in turn triggers the coagulation cascade in the intrinsic pathway (factors XII, XI, IX and VIII – listed in the order they are stimulated). This then triggers the final common pathway. Consequently, the activated partial thromboplastin time will become prolonged if there is a deficiency in any of the clotting factors in the intrinsic pathway (factors VIII, IX, XI and XII) or in the final common pathway (factors I, II, V and X). While this is a less accurate representation of the role of the intrinsic pathway *in vivo* – where it depends on thrombin generated by the tissue factor pathway – this test is still a simple and effective method for screening for potential clotting factor defects in the intrinsic and final common pathways.

Anticoagulant factors

There are also three anticoagulant proteins (protein C, protein S and antithrombin) that inhibit the coagulation cascade, shown in Figure 13.8. In normal conditions, these anticoagulant factors prevent the blood from coagulating inappropriately, allowing normal blood flow. When there is endothelial damage, triggering the clotting cascade, the anticoagulant factors

Figure 13.8 Anticoagulant proteins and the coagulation factors they inhibit. Arrows represent activation and flat lines represent inhibition. aPC, activated protein C; PC, protein C; PS, protein S; TF, tissue factor; TM, thrombomodulin.

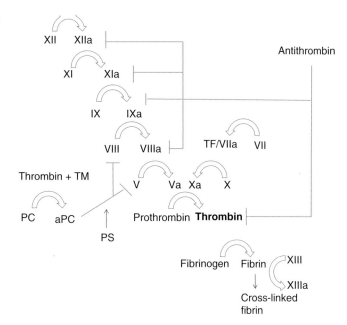

Figure 13.8 Anticoagulant proteins and the coagulation factors they inhibit. Arrows represent activation and flat lines represent inhibition. aPC, activated protein C; PC, protein C; PS, protein S; TF, tissue factor; TM, thrombomodulin.

are overcome by the clotting cascade, allowing a fibrin clot to form. Defects in these natural anticoagulants are important as hereditary thrombophilias (see also Chapter 14).

Fibrinolysis

After haemostasis has been achieved, the body has a mechanism for the enzymatic lysis of clots. In fibrinolysis, plasminogen is converted into plasmin, an enzyme which causes lysis of fibrin clots. Activators of fibrinolysis include tissue plasminogen activator (tPA) and urokinase plasminogen activator (uPA). Inhibitors of fibrinolysis include plasminogen activator inhibitor 1, α2-antiplasmin and thrombin activatable fibrinolysis inhibitor 1. Following the lysis of fibrin, fibrin degradation products such as D-dimers are released (Figure 13.9).

In life-threatening pulmonary embolism (and other conditions such as acute ischaemic stroke or

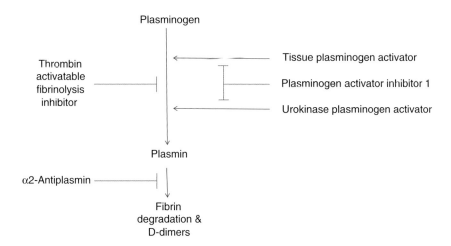

Figure 13.9 Normal fibrinolysis. Red arrows represent promoters of fibrinolysis and flat blue lines represent fibrinolysis inhibitors.

myocardial infarction), rapid lysis of the thrombosis may be needed and this is achieved through pharmacological activation of the fibrinolytic pathway. Thrombolytic drugs include urokinase (uPA) and recombinant tPA (alteplase, reteplase and tenecteplase) as well as non-physiological activators, such as streptokinase, derived from certain streptococci. Streptokinase binds to plasminogen and streptokinase-plasminogen complex activates free plasminogen. Fibrinolysis may be inhibited by antifibrinolytic drugs such as tranexamic acid, which are used to reduce perioperative bleeding when moderate to high volumes of blood loss are expected, or in major bleeding.

Congenital (inherited) disorders of the coagulation system

Blood clotting abnormalities can be divided into two categories: congenital and acquired defects. This section deals with those inherited disorders (Table 13.2) that are present from birth: haemophilia A and haemophilia B.

The term *haemophilia*, first used by Schönlein in 1839, was applied to a lifelong tendency to prolonged haemorrhage found in males and dependent on the transmission of a sex-linked abnormal gene. During the decade 1950–1960, it was found that there are in fact two diseases within the group of patients who, on clinical and genetic grounds, had been diagnosed as having haemophilia: patients with factor VIII deficiency and those with factor IX deficiency.

Haemophilia A (factor VIII deficiency): genetics and prevalence

Deficiency of factor VIII results from an abnormality in the factor VIII gene, a large gene (186 kilobases, 26 exons) lying at the tip of the long arm of the X chromosome. Various abnormalities in the nucleotide sequence of this gene have been identified, ranging from single-point mutations to large deletions, but half of all severe cases are caused by an inversion involving intron 22. The disease is almost entirely confined to hemizygous males, because the normal X chromosome in heterozygous females is almost always capable of bringing about adequate factor VIII production. The prevalence of this disorder is about one per 10 000 males. Females with haemophilia have been observed extremely rarely and these are either homozygotes for the abnormal gene or are heterozygotes in whom the normal X chromosome has not produced sufficient quantities of factor VIII because of lyonization.

Daughters of males with haemophilia are obligatory carriers of the gene, because they must inherit the abnormal X chromosome. Sons, on the other hand, will not inherit the haemophilia gene, because they inherit the Y chromosome. A female with a genetic defect on one X chromosome will transmit the disease to half of her sons, and half of her daughters will become carriers. Patients suspected of having haemophilia should be carefully questioned for a history of a bleeding disorder occurring in relations on the maternal side as opposed to the paternal side. There is a steady spontaneous mutation rate of the gene responsible for factor VIII production, because approximately one-third of all people with haemophilia have no family history of the disease; this has been corroborated by studies on the genomic DNA.

Detection of carriers and antenatal diagnosis

On average, female carriers have half of the FVIII clotting activity compared to normal; however, a normal FVIII level does not exclude carrier status, and genetic mutational analysis is required.

Table 13.2 **A summary of common inherited bleeding disorders and their treatments.**

	Severe haemophilia A	Mild haemophilia A	Von Willebrand disease
Inheritance	X-linked recessive	X-linked recessive	Most commonly autosomal dominant
Pattern of bleeding	Spontaneous joint and muscle bleeding	Bleeding following trauma or surgery	Mucocutaneous bleeding
Mechanism	Severe deficiency of factor VIII	Mild deficiency of factor VIII	Deficiency of von Willebrand factor
Treatment	Prophylactic treatment with recombinant factor VIII or emicizumab	On-demand treatment with factor VIII	On-demand treatment with DDAVP® or von Willebrand factor-containing concentrates

Prenatal diagnosis of haemophilia can be made by analysis of fetal DNA, which can be obtained either by chorionic villus sampling between 11.5 and 14 weeks gestation or by amniocentesis after 16 weeks. Invasive prenatal diagnosis techniques are associated with a risk of miscarriage. In some cases, a late amniocentesis (at 34–36 weeks) is performed to avoid the risk of miscarriage and to give advance notice of the diagnosis before delivery.

Clinical features

The characteristic clinical feature of severe haemophilia is the occurrence of spontaneous bleeding into the joints (Figure 13.10) and, less frequently, the muscles; these two sites account for about 95% of all bleeds requiring treatment. The presenting symptom is pain in the affected area and this can be very severe. People with haemophilia rapidly become expert at diagnosing the onset of haemorrhage in its earliest stages, allowing treatment with recombinant factor VIII infusion to be initiated at a time when it can be most effective. If not properly treated, bleeding into joints results in long-term joint dysfunction. The knees, elbows and ankles are most commonly affected. Haematuria, epistaxis and gastrointestinal bleeding are less common. Intracranial bleeding is the most common cause of death from the disease itself, accounting for 25–30% of all such deaths; only about half of the affected patients have a history of trauma.

The severity of bleeding and mode of presentation are related to the level of plasma factor VIII. In severe haemophilia (FVIII <0.01 IU/mL) spontaneous bleeds occur, in moderately severe haemophilia (FVIII 0.01–0.05 IU/mL) there is only very occasional spontaneous bleeding but severe bleeding can occur after minor trauma, and in mild haemophilia (FVIII >0.05 to <0.4 IU/mL) bleeding usually only occurs after trauma. The severity of the disease often remains consistent throughout a family.

Because of treatment with HIV-contaminated factor VIII concentrates between about 1978 and 1985, over 50% of patients with severe haemophilia in the USA and Europe became HIV positive; many of these have died of the acquired immune deficiency syndrome (AIDS). In addition, many people treated for severe haemophilia before 1985 were infected with hepatitis C virus, before formal identification of this virus and the use of virally inactivated factor concentrates. The majority of patients are now treated with recombinant factor VIII which does not convey a risk of infection.

Approximately 25% of patients with haemophilia A develop antibodies that inhibit the functional activity of the factor concentrate. These can make haemophilia more challenging to treat and increase the risk of bleeding.

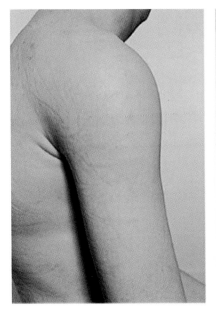
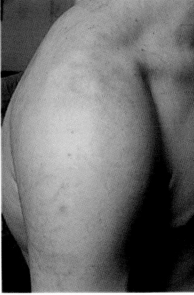

Figure 13.10 Haemarthrosis of the shoulder joint in a patient with haemophilia A.

Diagnosis

The possibility of haemophilia is suggested by the combination of appropriate clinical features (with or without a relevant family history) and the finding of a normal PT and a prolonged APTT. Confirmation is by a specific assay of factor VIII coagulant activity. vWD must also be excluded because of vWF's role as a carrier for factor VIII.

Treatment

Patients with severe haemophilia are offered prophylactic treatment in infancy to prevent bleeding. Standard treatment is with regular intravenous factor VIII replacement. Patients (or their parents/guardians) are taught how to administer this intravenously at home. Historically, the factor VIII used to be a plasma-derived high-purity factor VIII concentrate. Now patients are treated with recombinant factor VIII, which is not a plasma product so is not associated with a risk of viral transmission. The aim of prophylactic treatment is to keep the patient's factor VIII level above 0.01 IU/mL. Factor VIII is often required every 48 hours to maintain this trough level.

More recently, extended half-life factor VIII has moved into clinical practice. The recombinant factor VIII is linked to another molecule that causes it to be retained in the circulation for longer. The other molecules include polyethylene glycol (PEG), Fc fusion proteins and albumin. The treatment strategy with extended half-life factor VIII products is similar but dosing intervals can be spaced out more.

Other strategies for the treatment of haemophilia A relate to an understanding of the normal role of factor VIII, which is responsible for linking factor IX and X into close enough proximity for factor X to become activated. Emicizumab, a bispecific antibody that links activated factor IX to factor X, mimics this action and has the advantage that it can be given subcutaneously every 1–4 weeks. Further advances include gene therapies which introduce the missing factor VIII gene into the liver, where it can be induced to form factor VIII. Gene therapies are still at the research stage at present and are not in widespread use.

For patients with mild or moderate haemophilia A, regular prophylactic treatment is not usually needed, although in some cases of moderate haemophilia A associated with bleeding complications, this may be needed. Recombinant factor VIII treatment is given on demand to treat spontaneous or post-traumatic bleeding, and is also often required before surgery to prevent bleeding.

For people with haemophilia and inhibitors, haemorrhage may require treatment with 'bypassing agents' such as recombinant factor VIIa or FEIBA (factor eight inhibitor bypassing activity; that is, a plasma-derived activated prothrombin complex concentrate), which activate the coagulation cascade without requiring factor VIII. Emicizumab has also proven effective for patients with inhibitors because it bypasses factor VIII.

Haemophilia B (factor IX deficiency, Christmas disease)

The clinical features and inheritance of factor IX deficiency, haemophilia B, are identical to those in factor VIII deficiency, with haemophilia B being the less common condition. The factor IX gene is located on the long arm of the X chromosome and is much smaller than the factor VIII gene (containing eight exons). Mutations in this gene have been found in virtually all cases of factor IX deficiency.

As with haemophilia A, the APTT will be prolonged and the PT normal. The diagnosis can be made by assay of the factor IX level. Treatment is aimed at maintaining the factor IX level above 0.01 IU/mL, and this is accomplished with recombinant factor IX products administered approximately every 3 days. Extended half-life products have produced recombinant factor IX concentrates with dramatically extended half-lives, allowing haemophilia B patients to receive prophylaxis with a single injection per week. Gene therapy has been used for haemophilia B and remains under active investigation. Inhibitors to infused factor IX are rare.

Deficiency of other clotting factors

Single deficiencies of factors other than VIII and IX are rare, but all possible deficiencies have been found and all except factor XII deficiency may give rise to bleeding disorders of varying degrees of severity. The explanation for the absence of excessive haemorrhage in factor XII deficiency is that the physiological activator of factor IX is thrombin, not factor XII.

Acquired coagulation disorders

Patients with advanced liver disease often have several abnormalities in haemostasis, since the hepatocyte is the major cell type involved in the synthesis of most of the coagulation factors. Factor VIII is produced in liver sinusoidal cells, however, and while other factors are

Table 13.3 The multiple haemostatic defects in severe liver disease lead to a precarious rebalancing of haemostasis.

Predisposing towards bleeding	Predisposing towards thrombosis
↓ Fibrinogen	↑ Factor VIII
↓ Factors II, V, VII, IX, X, XI, XIII	↑ Von Willebrand factor
↓ Platelets	↓ Protein C
↑ Tissue plasminogen activator	↓ Protein S
↑ Urokinase plasminogen activator	↓ Antithrombin
↓ α2-Antiplasmin	↓ ADAMTS13
↓ Thrombin activatable fibrinolysis inhibitor	↑ Plasminogen activator inhibitor 1

usually deficient, factor VIII is often elevated in liver disease. The anticoagulant factors (protein C, protein S and antithrombin) are also produced by the liver. The deficiency of both procoagulant and anticoagulant factors leads to a precarious rebalancing of haemostasis (Table 13.3). Patients with severe liver disease will often have a prolonged PT but this does not necessarily correlate with bleeding risk because it does not take the deficiency of anticoagulant factors into account. Bleeding risk for patients with severe liver disease is more closely associated with portal venous pressure and the presence of oesophageal varices.

The final stages in the synthesis of factors II, VII, IX and X involve a vitamin K-dependent carboxylase, which adds carboxyl (-COOH) groups to the proteins; these groups are necessary for the efficient functioning of the molecules. In warfarin therapy (see Chapter 14), this process is inhibited, leading to deficiencies in these factors.

Similar abnormalities are seen in vitamin K deficiency, which may be found in the newborn (haemorrhagic disease of the newborn), in patients with intestinal malabsorption and, because bile salts are required for vitamin K absorption, also in patients with biliary obstruction or biliary fistulae. Vitamin K deficiency may be corrected with vitamin K replacement.

Disseminated intravascular coagulation

Disseminated intravascular coagulation (DIC) describes a process in which there is inappropriate generalized activation of the clotting system with simultaneous marked activation of the fibrinolytic system. DIC does not occur on its own and is always due to an underlying condition. Patients with DIC are often severely unwell. In pregnancy, acute DIC may be associated with premature separation of the placenta (placental abruption), amniotic fluid embolism or shock. DIC may also be seen in certain bacterial infections such as meningococcal septicaemia, where the endotoxin causes damage to monocytes and vascular endothelium. It is a common complication following intravascular haemolysis of red cells after a mismatched transfusion. The syndrome also occurs occasionally after extensive trauma, brain injury, extensive burns or snake bites. Chronic DIC may occur due to disseminated carcinoma and some haematological malignancies (especially acute promyelocytic leukaemia, see Chapter 8).

In those diseases that are associated with DIC, the clotting cascade may be activated by expression of tissue factor on damaged tissues or activated monocytes or by abnormal activators of coagulation. Activation of the cascade leads to the generation and dissemination of large amounts of thrombin in the circulation, the activation of platelets and the formation of intravascular microthrombi. If this is sufficiently extensive, there is a reduction of the concentration of fibrinogen and other clotting factors in the plasma, which impairs haemostatic activity. As a consequence of the fibrin formation, the fibrinolytic mechanism is activated, resulting in high concentrations of fibrin degradation products, including D-dimers.

The haemorrhagic manifestations may be so severe in acute DIC as to lead to death. They include petechiae, ecchymoses and bleeding from the nose, mouth, urinary and gastrointestinal tracts and vagina. Haemorrhage may also occur into the pituitary gland, liver, adrenals and brain.

Although the usual clinical manifestation of acute DIC is haemorrhage, occasionally the clinical picture is dominated by signs and symptoms of widespread thrombosis and infarction. Thrombi are most frequently found in the microvasculature; there may be digital gangrene, adult respiratory distress syndrome, neurological signs and renal failure. Mild hypotension is commonly present in acute DIC and may progress to become more severe and irreversible if not treated in time.

In chronic DIC, the haemorrhagic tendency may be mild or moderate. However, some patients with chronic DIC are asymptomatic because the activation of the clotting and fibrinolytic systems is finely balanced and the production of clotting factors and platelets is sufficiently increased to compensate for their increased consumption.

Diagnosis

This is partly dependent on being aware of the conditions with which DIC is associated. The investigations of value in the diagnosis of acute or chronic DIC are as follows (Table 13.4).

- *Platelet count.* Platelets become enmeshed in the fibrin clots on the vascular endothelium and thrombocytopenia is an early and common sign.
- *APTT and PT.* These are usually prolonged, because of the depletion of clotting factors, especially in acute DIC.
- *Fibrinogen concentration.* This is usually reduced as fibrinogen is consumed into the thrombi.
- *D-dimers.* D-dimers are increased because of increased fibrinolysis.

Treatment

Treatment should always be aimed at treating the underlying cause, for instance, treating any underlying sepsis. The clotting derangements seen in DIC do not usually need treatment in themselves as long as there is no clinically evident thrombosis or bleeding. However, in the presence of bleeding, or invasive procedures that may result in bleeding, treatment with platelet transfusions, plasma and cryoprecipitate may be required (to correct thrombocytopenia, clotting factor deficiencies and fibrinogen deficiencies respectively). When patients with DIC develop thrombosis, cautious anticoagulation is required, as patients will also have an elevated risk of bleeding.

Table 13.4 Summary of laboratory findings for investigation of bleeding disorders.

	Platelet count	Platelet function	PT	APTT	Factor VIII	Factor IX	Von Willebrand factor
Thrombocytopenia	↓	↔	↔	↔	↔	↔	↔
Platelet function disorder	↔	↓	↔	↔	↔	↔	↔
Haemophilia A	↔	↔	↔	↑	↓	↔	↔
Haemophilia B	↔	↔	↔	↑	↔	↓	↔
Von Willebrand disease	↔	↓/↔	↔	↑/↔	↓/↔	↔	↓

APTT, activated partial thromboplastin time; PT, prothrombin time.

14

Thrombosis and anticoagulant therapy

LEARNING OBJECTIVES

After reading this chapter, you should be able to:

✔ outline the diagnosis of deep vein thrombosis and pulmonary embolism

✔ describe venous anatomy for classification of deep vein thrombosis

✔ understand the principles of anticoagulant therapy with unfractionated heparin, low molecular weight heparin, warfarin and the direct oral anticoagulants

✔ describe the natural anticoagulant mechanisms in blood and some of the prothrombotic states (thrombophilias)

✔ recognize the risk of thrombosis in pregnancy.

Venous thromboembolism

While Chapter 13 examined the haemostatic system with a view to understanding disorders leading to bleeding, disorders also arise which cause excessive or inappropriate clotting. The disorders of venous thromboembolism include deep vein thromboses and pulmonary emboli, as well as more unusual venous thromboses such as cerebral venous sinus thrombosis or splanchnic vein thrombosis. The incidence of venous thrombosis is 1–2 per 1000 people in the United Kingdom per year.

In deep vein thrombosis, a thrombus obstructs one of the deep vessels of the leg (or, less commonly, arm), limiting venous return. This may lead to symptoms of swelling, pain, redness or warmth in the affected limb.

Pulmonary embolism is due to thrombosis occluding one of the pulmonary arteries (or one of their branches). Occlusion of the pulmonary artery reduces oxygen transfer from the lungs into the circulation, leading to hypoxia. The severity of symptoms is usually proportionate to the size of the thrombosis and the suddenness of its onset. Symptoms may include breathlessness, pleuritic chest pain, presyncope, syncope and sudden death. Pulmonary emboli are usually the consequence of a deep vein thrombosis, where part of the thrombosis breaks away, travelling through the venous system until it reaches the pulmonary vasculature and occludes one of the pulmonary arteries. Venous thromboembolism may arise as a complication of hospital treatment for other conditions and is the leading cause of avoidable hospital care associated mortality in the UK.

Haematology Lecture Notes, Eleventh Edition. Deborah Hay, Andrew King and Michael Desborough.
© 2023 John Wiley & Sons Ltd. Published 2023 by John Wiley & Sons Ltd.
Companion website: www.wiley.com/go/Hay/Haematology/11e

Virchow's triad and risk factors for venous thromboembolism

There are three broad groups of risk factors for developing venous thromboembolism. These groups comprise Virchow's triad: venous stasis, endothelial damage and hypercoagulability (Table 14.1).

To reduce the risk of venous thromboembolism, hospitalized patients are encouraged to mobilize early and to keep hydrated. Chemical thromboprophylaxis, usually with prophylactic low molecular weight heparin (see below), is used to reduce the thrombosis risk. Mechanical measures such as antiembolic stockings or intermittent pneumatic compression devices may also be used to increase venous return to reduce the risk of thrombosis.

Table 14.1 Virchow's triad and examples of risk factors for venous thromboembolism.

Component of Virchow's triad	Clinical examples of prothrombotic disorder
Venous stasis	Prolonged immobility (e.g. long-haul flights, long-term bed rest, paraplegia) Postoperative (especially abdominal, pelvic or orthopaedic) Obstruction of venous return (e.g. gravid uterus, pelvic or inguinal lymphadenopathy)
Endothelial damage	Trauma, sepsis, chronic inflammation
Hypercoagulability	Pregnancy, combined oral contraceptive pill Cancer Inherited deficiency of natural anticoagulants. protein C and S, and antithrombin; or mutations in procoagulant factors (e.g. factor V Leiden, prothrombin gene mutation) Antiphospholipid syndrome

Venous anatomy and the clinical presentation of venous thromboembolism

It is important to distinguish thrombosis in deep veins from those in superficial veins, and thrombosis in proximal deep veins from thrombosis in distal deep veins. These conditions have different treatments. Proximal veins in the leg include any vein proximal to the popliteal fossa. This includes the popliteal vein, femoral vein, superficial femoral vein (which, despite its name, is not a superficial vein), common femoral vein, external iliac vein, internal iliac vein and vena cava. Proximal thromboses are at the greatest risk of breaking apart and causing pulmonary emboli. Distal veins include all veins distal to the popliteal fossa, including the peroneal veins, anterior tibial vein, posterior tibial vein and gastrocnemius veins. Distal thromboses are unlikely to break away to form pulmonary emboli so anticoagulation treatment does not need to be as intensive (Figure 14.1).

Superficial veins in the lower limb include the long and short saphenous veins. Thromboses within these veins are often painful but are at low risk of forming pulmonary emboli. The exception to this are thromboses that are protruding through the saphenofemoral junction (the meeting between the superficial and deep venous systems) and these are classified as deep vein thromboses. Deep vein thrombosis should be suspected clinically in a patient with unilateral leg pain or swelling that is otherwise unexplained.

The pulmonary arteries start as a trunk and then bifurcate into a left and right main trunk. These veins branch into lobar branches, then segmental branches, then subsegmental branches. Pulmonary emboli occluding the larger vessels are more likely to lead to severe symptoms such as syncope, hypotension and sudden death. Smaller pulmonary emboli will be more likely to present as pleuritic chest pain or breathlessness on exertion.

Diagnosis of venous thromboembolism

As the features of deep vein thrombosis (DVT) especially are relatively common (for example, due to cellulitis of the leg), clinical scoring systems have

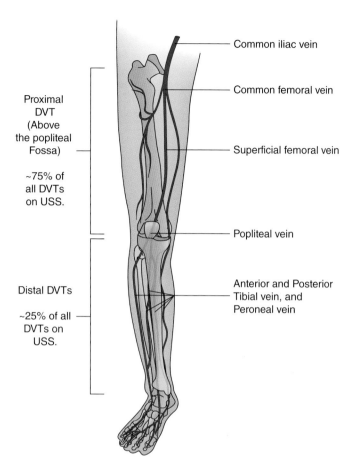

Figure 14.1 Venous anatomy and the clinical presentation of venous thromboembolism.

Common iliac vein

Common femoral vein

Proximal DVT (Above the popliteal Fossa)

~75% of all DVTs on USS.

Superficial femoral vein

Popliteal vein

Distal DVTs

~25% of all DVTs on USS.

Anterior and Posterior Tibial vein, and Peroneal vein

been developed to assess the likelihood of a venous thrombosis and to guide further diagnostic testing. In the UK, the Wells score is used to assess the risk of thrombosis. The Wells scores for DVT and pulmonary embolism are different (Table 14.2). Patients considered at high risk of venous thromboembolism from the Wells score will proceed directly to imaging. For patients considered to be at low risk using the Wells score, a D-dimer test may be used to further stratify the risk. A patient with low risk on the Wells score and a normal D-dimer does not need further imaging as the risk of venous thromboembolism is low. A patient with low risk on the Wells score and an elevated D-dimer should proceed to further imaging. Clinical judgement should be used in each case.

Imaging for a DVT will usually be with compression ultrasonography of the affected leg (or arm). Imaging for pulmonary emboli is most commonly performed using CT pulmonary angiography or ventilation/perfusion scans. Since there is a high risk of a venous thromboembolism worsening if untreated, anticoagulation should start as soon as a DVT or pulmonary embolism is suspected and can be stopped if a venous thromboembolism is excluded.

Treatment of venous thromboembolism

First-line treatment for proximal DVT or pulmonary emboli is with anticoagulant drugs, of which several

Table 14.2 **Wells score for risk stratification for deep vein thrombosis (DVT) and pulmonary embolism (PE).**

Wells score feature	For potential deep vein thrombosis	For potential pulmonary embolism
Active cancer	+1	+1
Recent surgery or immobilization	+1	+1
Previous DVT (or PE)	+1	+1.5
Calf swelling 3 cm or more compared to asymptomatic calf	+1	N/A
Collateral superficial veins	+1	N/A
Pitting oedema confined to the symptomatic leg	+1	N/A
Swelling of entire leg	+1	N/A
Localized tenderness along distribution of deep venous system	+1	N/A
Paralysis, paresis or recent cast immobilization of lower extremities	+1	N/A
Haemoptysis	N/A	+1
Heart rate more than 100 beats per minute	N/A	+1.5
Clinical signs of DVT	N/A	+3
Alternative diagnosis at least as likely as DVT (or PE)	−2	−3
Final score	**2+ points:** **DVT likely** **Proceed to compression ultrasonography**	**5+ points:** **PE likely** **Proceed to computed tomography pulmonary angiogram**
	One point or less: DVT unlikely; proceed to D-dimer for risk stratification	Four points or less: PE unlikely; proceed to D-dimer for risk stratification

are available, including warfarin and the direct-acting anticoagulants (see below). In the majority of situations, direct oral anticoagulants have a similar efficacy to warfarin and may have a lower risk of bleeding. The main risk from each anticoagulant is of bleeding but in the acute treatment phase, the benefits of anticoagulation considerably outweigh the risks.

The initial duration of anticoagulation is usually 3–6 months (most commonly 3 months). Beyond this, a risk assessment should be made about the risk of another thrombosis if anticoagulation is stopped and this should be balanced against the risk of bleeding on anticoagulation.

For pulmonary emboli and proximal deep vein thromboses that have a strong provoking factor, for instance recent major surgery, the risk of recurrent

thrombosis is relatively low. Consequently, the risk of bleeding from anticoagulation outweighs the risk of recurrent thrombosis and it is usually stopped after 3 months. However, for unprovoked venous thromboembolism (that is to say, where no provoking factors have been identified), the risk of recurrent thrombosis is considerably higher (approximately 7.5–10% per year for men, 3–5% per year for women) and the risk and benefits of long-term anticoagulation should be assessed. Distal deep vein thromboses, with their lower risk of embolization, are usually anticoagulated for only short periods of time, and superficial thromboses may need no therapeutic anticoagulation at all.

Rarely, catheter-directed thrombolysis with or without venous stenting may also be considered for DVT.

This is indicated in circumstances where the affected limb is severely compromised with symptoms of phlegmasia. In some centres, it may also be considered for those with large proximal venous thrombosis.

Patients with acute DVT who are considered to be at high risk of bleeding and who cannot receive anticoagulants may be considered for a temporary inferior vena cava filter. The filter is placed in the inferior vena cava by an interventional radiologist such that it will prevent pulmonary embolism by catching thromboemboli from deep vein thromboses that break off and travel up the vena cava. Since they are in themselves potentially prothrombotic, these filters should be placed for the minimum possible duration of time and then removed, and should only be used in exceptional cases.

Patients with life-threatening pulmonary emboli may be considered for systemic or catheter-directed thrombolytic therapy with thrombolytic agents such as alteplase, tenecteplase or urokinase. These medications rapidly lyse the thrombus but at the risk of significant major bleeding. In cases at the highest risk of bleeding with life-threatening pulmonary emboli, surgical thrombectomy may be considered.

At present, all patients with pulmonary emboli should be considered for anticoagulation. There is controversy over whether subsegmental pulmonary emboli (the smallest emboli) always require treatment and ongoing clinical trials may help to resolve this question.

Complications of venous thromboembolism

The most life-threatening risk from a deep vein thrombosis is that it may break away and cause a pulmonary embolism. This risk is highest in the first month after diagnosis (approximately 40% if anticoagulation is not given) and remains high for months 2 and 3 after diagnosis (approximately 10% per month if anticoagulation is not given). Beyond the first 3 months, the risk of a pulmonary embolism falls substantially.

Pulmonary emboli may have long-term complications. Chronic thromboembolic pulmonary hypertension occurs in approximately 2% of patients post PE. It may cause chronic breathlessness and increases the risk of mortality. It is caused by chronic thrombosis leading to reduced oxygen transfer and to subsequent increases in pulmonary artery pressure in an attempt to compensate for the reduced perfusion. It is diagnosed by demonstrating chronic thromboemboli on a CT pulmonary angiogram or ventilation/perfusion scan, and through demonstrating elevated pulmonary artery pressures, usually with an echocardiogram or through right heart catheterization. Treatments include medications to relax the pulmonary vasculature and surgical treatments such as pulmonary endarterectomy.

Deep vein thrombosis itself may also have long-term complications. DVTs may lead to post-thrombotic syndrome, a chronic problem caused by damage to the affected veins and/or venous valves. Post-thrombotic syndrome occurs in 23–60% of patients who have had a DVT and usually occurs within 2 years of diagnosis. Symptoms include a feeling of heaviness in the leg, itching, tingling or cramping, swelling in the leg and discolouration of the skin. When symptoms are mild, no treatment is indicated. Some patients find that well-fitted below-knee compression stockings reduce their symptoms. In the most severe cases, venous stenting may be considered to relieve symptoms.

Thrombosis and the COVID-19 pandemic

During the COVID-19 pandemic starting in late 2019, it became apparent that patients with severe COVID-19 infection had a higher rate of venous thrombosis than would be expected for people with a similar level of illness. Some of these thromboses were due to classic risk factors such as immobility and inflammation. However, there was also an increase in small segmental and subsegmental pulmonary emboli without evidence of deep vein thrombosis. These have been termed *immunothromboses* and are thought to arise from inflammation of the pulmonary vasculature rather than from deep vein thromboses breaking away to form pulmonary emboli. The pathological basis of these immunothromboses and whether they need different treatment from classic pulmonary emboli are still topics of debate.

There has also been a risk of an exceptionally rare thrombotic syndrome following COVID-19 vaccination using adenoviral vaccines such as the ChAdOx1 nCoV-19 vaccine. This has been termed *vaccine-induced thrombosis and thrombocytopenia* (VITT). VITT is due to antibodies forming against platelet factor 4 leading to formation of thromboses. This has a similar mechanism to heparin-induced thrombotic thrombocytopenia. VITT has often manifested as cerebral venous sinus thromboses associated with thrombocytopenia and has been challenging to treat. The mainstay of treatment has been anticoagulation and intravenous immunoglobulin. The risk of death of thrombosis from COVID-19 infection remains very much higher than the small risks from the vaccines.

Anticoagulant drugs

Anticoagulant drugs are widely used for the treatment and prophylaxis of venous thromboembolism in a range of clinical settings. The main anticoagulant drugs are heparin (including unfractionated heparin and low molecular weight heparin), vitamin K antagonists such as warfarin, and the direct oral anticoagulants (DOACs) (Table 14.3). Heparins do not cross the placenta and are therefore preferred when anticoagulation is required during pregnancy.

Heparin

Heparin is a mixture of glycosaminoglycan chains extracted from porcine mucosa. Unfractionated heparin (UFH) chains average 15 000 Da while low molecular weight heparin (LMWH) is a mixture of smaller chains averaging 5000 Da. All heparins depend on a specific pentasaccharide sequence for binding to antithrombin. UFH is usually administered intravenously, when its biological half-life is 1–2 hours – this makes it useful in clinical situations where short-term control of the degree of anticoagulation is essential. LMWH is given by subcutaneous injection once or twice daily, and is commonly used for inpatient thromboprophylaxis.

Heparin potentiates the action of antithrombin, leading to inactivation of the activated serine protease coagulation factors thrombin (IIa) and Xa. Heparin chains longer than 18 saccharides in length can link antithrombin and IIa molecules, leading to powerful inhibition; shorter chains act predominantly by potentiating the action against Xa. Examples of LMWHs currently in use are dalteparin, enoxaparin and tinzaparin. Fondaparinux has a similar mechanism to LMWH but is a synthetic pentasaccharide that induces antithrombin specifically to inhibit Xa.

Table 14.3 Summary of commonly used anticoagulants.

	Unfractionated heparin	Low molecular weight heparin	Warfarin	Dabigatran	Apixaban, edoxaban and rivaroxaban
Mechanism	Inhibition of factor Xa and IIa (and also IXa and XIa) by binding to antithrombin	Inhibition of factor Xa by binding to antithrombin	Inhibition of vitamin K-dependent factors (II, VII, IX, X)	Inhibition of thrombin (factor IIa)	Inhibition of factor Xa
Half-life	1–2 hours	3–7 hours	4–5 days	12–18 hours	Apixaban 12 hours Edoxaban 10–14 hours Rivaroxaban 7–11 hours
Route of administration	Intravenous infusion	Subcutaneous	Oral	Oral	Oral
Monitoring	Activated partial thromboplastin time (APTT) or anti-factor Xa levels	Not routinely needed Anti-factor Xa levels	International normalized ratio (INR)	Not routinely needed Dilute thrombin time or ecarin clotting time (calibrated for dabigatran)	Not routinely needed Anti-factor Xa assay (calibrated for individual drug)
Reversal agent	Protamine sulfate	Protamine sulfate	Vitamin K and prothrombin complex concentrate	Idaracizumab	Andexanet alpha (prothrombin complex concentrate and tranexamic acid may be used when andexanet not available)

LMWH heparin is usually given in preference to UFH because its subcutaneous route of injection (rather than intravenous) and its stability (compared to UFH which needs regular monitoring) make it easier to use.

The anticoagulation intensity of UFH can be calculated using the activated partial thromboplastin time because it inhibits several factors within the intrinsic pathway. The activated partial thromboplastin time is not a reliable measure of LMWH. Both UFH and LMWH anticoagulation intensity may be measured by assessing inhibition of factor Xa.

Haemorrhage from overdosage is managed by stopping heparin and, if necessary, by giving protamine sulfate intravenously. UFH can be completely reversed by protamine, whereas LMWH is only partially reversed. Side-effects of heparin include heparin-induced thrombocytopenia (HIT) via an antibody-based mechanism, osteoporosis (following long-term use), alopecia and hypersensitivity reactions.

Warfarin

Warfarin is a coumarin derivative that is administered orally once a day, making it a convenient long-term outpatient anticoagulant. It is a vitamin K antagonist and interferes with post-translational carboxylation and hence with the functional activity of factors II, VII, IX and X (and the natural anticoagulants protein C and protein S).

Warfarin prolongs the prothrombin time and is usually monitored using the international normalized ratio (INR). To calculate the INR, the patient's prothrombin time is divided by the mean normal prothrombin time (calculated from testing normal volunteers). This is raised to the power of a correction factor (the international sensitivity index). The INR shows approximately how many times longer a patient's prothrombin time is compared to the normal population. For instance, an INR of 1 indicates that the patient's prothrombin time is the same as the normal population whereas an INR of 2 suggests the patient's prothrombin time is approximately double that of the normal population. A normal INR is approximately 0.8–1.2. For patients on warfarin or other vitamin K antagonists, the INR target is usually 2–3. For patients at particularly high risk of thrombosis, the INR target may be raised higher, most commonly to 3–4. The higher the INR, the greater the risk of bleeding.

One of the challenges of warfarin treatment is that there is wide inter-individual variation in response to a given dose of this drug, such that dosing needs to be tailored to each individual patient. There are also significant interactions between warfarin and other medications (as well as some foods and alcohol).

> **BOX 14.1 Emergency reversal of warfarin**
>
> In the event of major bleeding, rapid normalization of blood clotting will be required. Stopping warfarin will usually lead to a normal INR over 5–7 days – clearly too long a timescale in the event of significant ongoing or life-threatening haemorrhage. When faster normalization is needed then intravenous vitamin K will permit the γ-carboxylation of newly synthesized clotting factors, and will thereby reverse the effects of warfarin in 6–8 hours. This will still be too slow for the management of life-threatening bleeding, however.
>
> In this situation, prothrombin complex concentrate (PCC) is used. This product contains a mix of factors II, VII, IX and X and is therefore targeted exactly to the factors whose production is inhibited by warfarin. This PCC will reverse the effects of warfarin within minutes. The effect is not long-lived, however, and the INR will increase once the effect of the PCC wears off. For this reason, both PCC and vitamin K should be given at the same time in severe haemorrhage – the former to reverse the anticoagulant effect immediately, and the latter to ensure that synthesis of factors II, VII, IX and X is in place for when the effect of PCC is lost.

Together, these features mean that patients taking warfarin need to be monitored regularly with INR testing to ensure they have a consistent and appropriate degree of anticoagulation.

Warfarin may take several days to take effect, so LMWH is usually given alongside warfarin until the INR is consistently in the target range. As warfarin also reduces the natural anticoagulants protein C and protein S, patients may initially be relatively prothrombotic, so LMWH is essential in the first few days.

Warfarin crosses the placenta and may cause developmental abnormalities such as chondrodysplasia, microcephaly and blindness. It should therefore be avoided in the first trimester of pregnancy. It should also not be administered during the last few weeks of pregnancy because of its anticoagulant effect on the fetus and the consequent risk of fetal or placental haemorrhage.

For information on the emergency reversal of warfarin, see Box 14.1.

Direct oral anticoagulants (DOACs)

Orally available drugs that directly (i.e. without the involvement of antithrombin) inhibit either thrombin (dabigatran) or factor Xa (rivaroxaban, apixaban, edoxaban) have been developed.

All four drugs are an alternative to warfarin for the treatment and secondary prevention of venous thromboembolism and for stroke prevention in atrial fibrillation. For the treatment of acute venous thromboembolism, dabigatran and edoxaban require an initial 5 days of LMWH but rivaroxaban and apixaban do not. None of the drugs has a licence for prevention of embolic stroke and valve thrombosis in patients with mechanical heart valves.

One of the major advantages of DOACs in contrast to warfarin is that they are prescribed at fixed dose without the need for monitoring and dose adjustment. A rapid onset of action and short half-life also make initiation and interruption of anticoagulation considerably easier than with warfarin. Dabigatran levels can be measured using the dilute thrombin time or ecarin clotting time. In the event of major bleeding, dabigatran has a specific antidote (idarucizumab) that reverses its effect within minutes.

Anticoagulation intensity for the factor Xa inhibitors can be measured using an anti-factor Xa assay, calibrated to the individual drug. In the event of major bleeding, there is an antidote for factor Xa inhibitors (andexanet alfa) with a rapid onset of action. In the UK, this has currently only been approved for reversal of factor Xa inhibitors for patients with acute gastrointestinal bleeding. Further clinical trials are ongoing to assess andexanet alfa for reversal of anticoagulation in intracranial bleeding and before emergency surgery. Prothrombin complex may be used to reduce the effects of factor Xa inhibitors and is often given alongside tranexamic acid. This is not a reversal strategy but may reduce the anticoagulant effect.

Direct oral anticoagulants should not be prescribed in pregnancy or during breast feeding and women of child-bearing age should be warned of this.

Natural anticoagulant mechanisms and the prothrombotic state (thrombophilia)

As described in Chapter 13, there are natural anticoagulant mechanisms in the plasma that prevent localized fibrin formation from becoming widespread. The most important molecules involved in these mechanisms are antithrombin, protein C and protein S, all of which are produced in the liver. Inherited or acquired abnormalities of these inhibitors of coagulation may lead to a prothrombotic state (thrombophilia). This section summarizes the essential information relating to:

- the congenital deficiency of these factors
- prothrombotic states caused by the presence of a specific polymorphism in factor V (factor V Leiden) or prothrombin (G20210A polymorphism)
- an acquired prothrombotic state known as the antiphospholipid syndrome.

Antithrombin

This is mainly an inhibitor of thrombin and factor Xa, but it also inhibits factors IXa and XIa. Its action is markedly potentiated by heparin where antithrombin becomes activated by binding to endothelial cell-associated heparin sulfate and thus prevents thrombus formation on the endothelium. Congenital antithrombin deficiency, a form of inherited thrombophilia, is inherited in an autosomal dominant manner; its prevalence is about 1 in 3000. There are a number of molecular variants of antithrombin with different degrees of risk of thrombosis. Heterozygotes (whose antithrombin concentrations are 40–50% of normal) may develop recurrent DVT, mesenteric vein thrombosis and PE; the first thrombotic event usually occurs between the ages of 15 and 50 years.

Protein C and protein S

Two other inhibitors of coagulation are the vitamin K-dependent protein C and protein S. Protein C becomes activated (APC) when it reacts with thrombin bound to thrombomodulin, a protein of the endothelial cell membrane. APC is a serine protease that degrades factors Va and VIIIa in a reaction potentiated by its cofactor, protein S.

Some individuals have a hereditary deficiency of protein C, with about 50% of normal levels; these are heterozygotes for a mutation affecting the protein C gene and in one study were found with a prevalence of about 1 per 300. A proportion of such heterozygous individuals display the clinical picture seen in inherited antithrombin deficiency, but in addition are particularly prone to develop superficial thrombophlebitis, cerebral vein thrombosis and coumarin-induced skin necrosis. Homozygotes for the mutant gene are rare, and those who have virtually no protein C present with purpura fulminans or extensive thrombosis of visceral veins in the neonatal period.

The incidence of protein C deficiency in children and adults below the age of 45 years with recurrent venous thrombosis is about 5% and the incidence of protein S deficiency in this group is similar.

Factor V Leiden and APC resistance

A polymorphism in factor V at the APC cleavage site ($Arg^{506} \rightarrow Gln$) results in a factor Va molecule with resistance to degradation by APC. In white Caucasian populations, about 5% are heterozygous for this polymorphism, which is known as factor V Leiden (after its place of discovery). It is found in about 20% of cases of venous thrombosis. Heterozygotes have a 5–7-fold increase in the risk of thrombosis and homozygotes a 10–50-fold increase.

Prothrombin allele G20210A

Between 1% and 2% of the population have a G20210A polymorphism in the 3′ untranslated region of the prothrombin gene which leads to increased prothrombin levels. This increases the risk for venous thrombosis 2–4-fold.

Antiphospholipid syndrome

The antiphospholipid antibody syndrome is an acquired prothrombotic disorder defined by the presence of antiphospholipid antibodies (anticardiolipin antibodies, anti-β_2-glycoprotein I antibodies or lupus anticoagulant) and is associated with thrombosis or certain problems in pregnancy (recurrent early miscarriage, stillbirth and placental insufficiency).

Lupus anticoagulants prolong the results of coagulation tests that depend on phospholipid, and therefore have an apparent anticoagulant effect *in vitro*; however, they are associated with thromboses *in vivo*, due to the antibodies' effect on activating platelets and endothelial cells, as well as through more complex mechanisms. Features of the antiphospholipid syndrome therefore include recurrent venous thromboses (most commonly DVT of the lower limbs), recurrent arterial thrombosis (most commonly stroke) and recurrent miscarriage (caused by placental thrombosis and infarction). Thrombocytopenia may occur. Antiphospholipid antibodies are found in some patients with SLE or other autoimmune disorders as well as in individuals with no other evidence of an immunological abnormality.

Recent work on the mechanisms underlying the thrombotic tendency suggests that the relevant antibodies are those directed against P_2-glycoprotein I, these antibodies also being detected in the anticar-diolipin ELISA (β_2-glycoprotein I binds to negatively charged phospholipids) and in the lupus anticoagulant assay.

Patients with antiphospholipid syndrome are usually treated with warfarin (or other vitamin K antagonists) in preference to direct oral anticoagulants. Clinical trial evidence has suggested that particularly for patients with all three tests positive for antiphospholipid syndrome and for those with previous arterial thromboses, there is a lower risk for recurrent thrombosis with vitamin K antagonists than with direct oral anticoagulants.

Other causes of thrombosis

Paroxysmal nocturnal haemoglobinuria is described in Chapter 4. An important feature of this condition is an increased risk of venous and arterial thrombosis. While the mechanisms of thrombosis are incompletely understood, it is thought that complement-mediated intravascular cell lysis leads to the release of procoagulant microparticles into the circulation. While a rare cause of deep vein thrombosis or pulmonary embolism, paroxysmal nocturnal haemoglobinuria is a relatively more common cause of thrombosis in the splanchnic veins. Detection of paroxysmal nocturnal haemoglobinuria is important because it has a specific treatment: inhibition of the terminal complement cascade, with the anti-C5 monoclonal antibody eculizumab.

Myeloproliferative diseases are described in Chapter 8 and may also cause arterial and venous thromboses. They are often associated with splanchnic vein thrombosis. Treatment of venous thrombosis associated with myeloproliferative disease is with anticoagulation and with treatment of the underlying myeloproliferative disease.

Heparin-induced thrombotic thrombocytopenia is a condition where arterial and/or venous thromboses may form for patients taking heparin. The cause is an immune reaction between heparin and platelet factor 4, leading to the formation of platelet-rich clots. It usually occurs 5–10 days after starting heparin, although it may start within a day for patients who have previously had heparin, and is associated with a fall in the platelet count – often the first sign of concern clinically. Treatment is with cessation of heparin (and avoidance of this drug in future) and treatment with a non-heparin anticoagulant.

Venous thrombosis and pregnancy

The risk of venous thrombosis is substantially increased in pregnancy. This is due to a number of factors, including hormonally induced increased procoagulant proteins such as factor VIII and fibrinogen, decreased protein S, reduced mobility and pressure on the iliac veins from a gravid uterus. All pregnant women in the UK are assessed for risk of venous thromboembolism at their pregnancy booking appointment. For women considered at risk, prophylactic LMWH is given either antenatally and postnatally or just postnatally, depending on the calculated risk.

Diagnosis of venous thromboembolism in pregnancy may be challenging. Deep vein thrombosis of the legs may still be diagnosed with compression ultrasonography. However, this may miss thromboses within the proximal iliac veins. The diagnosis of pulmonary emboli is also more challenging because of the potential risk to the baby from ventilation/perfusion scans and to the mother's breast tissue (increased lifetime risk of breast cancer) from CT pulmonary angiography. The risks and benefits should be discussed with the mother when deciding on investigation and management strategies.

Warfarin and direct oral anticoagulants should not be used routinely in pregnancy because of actual or potential risks of teratogenicity. LMWH is the preferred treatment during pregnancy. Doses may need to be adjusted as pregnancy progresses. For pregnant women with antiphospholipid syndrome, aspirin should be considered in addition to LMWH.

15

Blood groups and blood transfusion

LEARNING OBJECTIVES

After reading this chapter, you should be able to:

✔ describe the inheritance and significance of the ABO blood group system

✔ describe the nature and significance of the Rh blood group system, including RhD

✔ explain the principles of the selection of donor blood of suitable ABO and Rh groups for a recipient, and the principles of the cross-match, including the antiglobulin test

✔ recognize the hazards of blood transfusion (incompatible blood, allergic reactions, bacterial infection, transmission of disease) and of massive blood transfusion

✔ investigate a patient suspected of receiving an incompatible transfusion

✔ outline the basis of blood fractionation and the rationale for the use of specific blood products, including red cells, platelet concentrates, fresh frozen plasma and cryoprecipitate

✔ describe the pathogenesis, clinical features and principles underlying the treatment and prevention of haemolytic disease of the newborn (HDN) caused by anti-D

✔ outline the principles of antenatal care concerned with predicting both the presence and severity of HDN caused by anti-D

✔ understand the differences between HDN caused by anti-D and that caused by anti-A and anti-B.

Blood transfusion and blood components

Many of the haematological disorders discussed in the preceding chapters result in anaemia and other cytopenias, or abnormalities of haemostasis. In addition, the treatment of these conditions frequently relies upon chemotherapy agents, which suppress bone marrow function. As a consequence, the transfusion of blood components forms a central pillar in the management of patients with haematological

---

Haematology Lecture Notes, Eleventh Edition. Deborah Hay, Andrew King and Michael Desborough.
© 2023 John Wiley & Sons Ltd. Published 2023 by John Wiley & Sons Ltd.
Companion website: www.wiley.com/go/Hay/Haematology/11e

disorders, and is also critically important in many other branches of medicine. Blood components available for transfusion include packed red cells, platelets, fresh frozen plasma, cryoprecipitate and granulocytes. Each of these products is discussed in further detail below, though we focus especially on packed red cells as the most widely transfused blood component.

Red cell transfusion

Packed red cells are the most widely used blood product. After donation of whole blood, most of the plasma is removed, leaving approximately 20 mL; a solution of saline with adenine, glucose and mannitol (SAG-M) is used to replace the rest of the plasma, and to maintain the viability of the red cells in storage. A unit of packed red cells is therefore typically ~300 mL in volume. It can be stored for 42 days at 4 °C. White cells are routinely removed from the red cell components through filtration (leucodepletion).

When to transfuse red cells

For patients who are anaemic and for whom transfusion is considered, it is important to consider treatable causes of anaemia such as iron deficiency, vitamin B12 deficiency or folate deficiency. The underlying cause of anaemia should be treated when possible in preference to red cell transfusion. For hospital inpatients who are not bleeding, red cell transfusion can be reserved for those whose haemoglobin concentration falls to 70 g/L or less, though this will not apply to patients with acute haemorrhage, where clinical judgement regarding transfusion is required. Individualized transfusion protocols are also needed for some groups such as those with acute coronary syndrome, who may require higher transfusion thresholds, or those on a chronic transfusion programme such as those with sickle cell disease.

For non-bleeding patients, a single unit of blood should be given at a time, followed by reassessment before further units to avoid overtransfusion. Such clinical guidelines are kept under regular revision by national transfusion specialists.

Alternatives to transfusion

Alternatives to blood transfusion should always be considered. As well as the simple correction of haematinics described above, erythropoietin may be considered in some patients to stimulate the bone marrow to produce more red cells. Other techniques may be used to minimize the amount of blood transfused, such as the use of tranexamic acid for surgery where significant blood loss is expected and for major bleeding. Perioperative cell salvage is a technique in which red cells lost due to bleeding during surgery can be filtered and returned to the patient, avoiding the need for donor blood transfusion.

Blood grouping and cross-matching

In order to permit safer transfusion, the donor blood group must be determined and the presence of antibodies established. Blood groups have arisen because of genetic divergence in the genes controlling the surface constituents of the red cells. The resulting alterations in the surface structures do not usually affect the function of the red cell, but when the red cells of a donor are transfused into a recipient who lacks these antigens, they may induce an immunological response, and an incompatible red cell transfusion may lead to acute haemolysis, renal failure, disseminated intravascular coagulation (DIC) and death.

There are 30 major blood group systems (e.g. ABO group, Rh group), together giving hundreds of possible red cell phenotypes. Although all the systems have given rise to transfusion difficulties (and indeed, this is how they have been recognized), this chapter focuses on the two of greatest importance: the ABO and Rh systems.

ABO system

Practically all red cells have the H antigen, a carbohydrate group attached mainly to proteins on the cell membrane. This antigen is the basis for the ABO blood groups. The ABO genetic locus is encoded on chromosome 9q, where one of three possible alleles may be found. The A allele encodes for a glycosyltransferase, which modifies the H antigen by adding N-acetylgalactosamine to it (thus forming the A antigen). The B allele of the ABO locus encodes an alternative glycosyltransferase that links galactose to the H antigen (thus converting it to the B antigen). The O allele, by contrast, encodes no functional enzyme at all, such that the H antigen remains unmodified. As each patient inherits an allele of the ABO locus on each copy of chromosome 9, there are six possible genotypes: AA, AO, BB, BO, AB and OO. As the O allele is non-functional, this means there are four possible phenotypes (known as ABO blood groups):

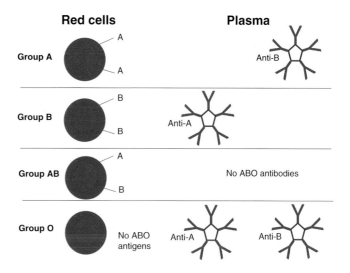

Figure 15.1 Red cell antigens and antibodies according to blood group. Anti-ABO blood group antibodies are IgM.

A, AB, B and O. The frequency of these ABO group phenotypes differs in different populations; in the UK the distribution is approximately 46% for group O, 42% for group A, 9% for group B and 3% for group AB.

Patients with group O blood (genotype OO) will have only unmodified H antigen on their red cells, but will have circulating immunoglobulin M (IgM) antibodies to the A and B antigens (Figure 15.1). These antibodies exist even if the patient has never been exposed to blood of another group; they are thought to arise as a result of cross-reactivity between the ABO antigens and commonly seen epitopes in bacteria and/or food products, because they are produced universally in the first year of life.

It is the naturally occurring presence of anti-A and/or anti-B antibodies that makes ABO typing so critical to blood transfusion practice. Transfusion of group A or B red cells to patients who have group O blood would result in binding of these preformed anti-A and anti-B antibodies to the transfused red cells, which would induce IgM-mediated intravascular haemolysis (see Chapter 4) – with the potential to cause renal failure, DIC and even death. Transfusion of group B blood to a patient of group A would have a similar effect but transfusing red cells from a donor with group O blood, featuring only the universal H antigen, should not produce a haemolytic response in patients of any ABO group. As such, group O has been termed the 'universal donor' group. While the 'universal donor' label is true to some extent, it is also subject to caveats: group O blood may not contain an ABO *antigen* that will cause haemolysis, but rarely blood from some group O donors will contain high-titre *antibodies* against groups A and B, which themselves might induce passive haemolysis of the recipient's own red cells. This must be borne in mind when determining safe donor blood groups for specific recipients.

Anti-A and anti-B antibodies will be found naturally in plasma. Thus, plasma from donors of blood group O will contain anti-A and anti-B, which could result in haemolysis if transfused into a recipient who has group A or B red cells. Thus, although group O donors are universal donors for red blood cells, their donated plasma must be given only to group O recipients (Table 15.1).

Rh system

The Rh system is also of great importance in transfusion medicine. It is frequently responsible for immunizing patients without the relevant Rh antigen, and can cause problems with both transfusion and pregnancy.

The inheritance of the Rh blood group system is more complex than that of the ABO system. Two separate genetic loci on chromosome 1 encode for a total of five antigens. The first locus, *RHD*, has alleles *D* or *d*; *D* encodes a transmembrane protein featuring the D antigen, while the allele *d* encodes a variant that does not bear this antigen. Patients are therefore considered to be RhD positive (the RhD antigen is their red cell surface) or RhD negative (they lack the RhD antigen). *RHCE* is an adjacent locus that encodes a transmembrane ion channel bearing the antigens *C* (or its variant, *c*) and *E* (or its variant, *e*). Alleles at this locus may be described as *CE*, *Ce*, *cE* or *ce*, denoting the set of antigens they encode. A complete description of the Rh haplotype for a patient will include

Table 15.1 ABO antigens and red cell or plasma transfusion. Donor red cells are only compatible if the recipient does not have antibodies against donor red cell antigens. If a recipient has antibodies against a donor ABO red cell antigen, this will lead to an acute haemolytic transfusion reaction. For plasma transfusion, an awareness of naturally occurring IgM antibodies in the donor plasma is essential.

Recipient blood group	Recipient antigens	Recipient antibodies	Safe donor blood groups for <u>red cell transfusion</u>	Safe donor blood groups for <u>plasma transfusion</u>
O	–	Anti-A Anti-B	O	O, A, B, AB
A	A	Anti-B	A or O	A, AB
B	B	Anti-A	B or O	B, AB
AB	A and B	–	AB, A, B or O	AB

alleles at both *RHD* and *RHCE* loci; for example, if a patient's full Rh genotype is DCe/DCE, they will have the *RhD* allele on both copies of chromosome 1, but *Ce* and *CE* alleles on the two different copies of chromosome 1 at the adjacent *RHCE* locus. They will therefore have the antigens D, C, E and e on their red cells.

The most common haplotypes are *DCe*, *dce* and *DcE*. The proximity of the two loci to each other means that meiotic crossing over is not seen, and the two loci are inherited as a unit.

The D antigen is the most clinically important of the Rh group antigens, because of its high immunogenicity. An RhD-negative person (e.g. genotype *dce/dce)* has a >50% chance of developing anti-D antibodies after the transfusion of one unit of RhD-positive red cells. By contrast, exposure to the c antigen will provoke anti-c production in only 2% of people lacking this antigen, such that the risk of immunization after giving red cells of type *dce/dce* to an individual who lacks the c antigen (for instance, a recipient with genotype *DCe/DCe)* is very small.

Note that unlike the ABO system, Rh antibodies are not naturally occurring; they must be raised by exposure of an antigen-negative individual to the appropriate antigen, either through transfusion of incompatible blood or through pregnancy (see section on haemolytic disease of the newborn, below). After the exposure, IgG antibodies come to predominate, and haemolysis is therefore generally extravascular (Figure 15.2).

Other blood group systems

Other blood group antibodies, which are sometimes a problem during blood transfusion, include the following: anti-K (Kell system), anti-Fyᵃ (Duffy system),

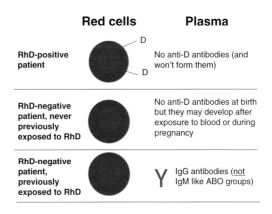

Red cells **Plasma**

RhD-positive patient — D / No anti-D antibodies (and won't form them) / D

RhD-negative patient, never previously exposed to RhD — No anti-D antibodies at birth but they may develop after exposure to blood or during pregnancy

RhD-negative patient, previously exposed to RhD — IgG antibodies (<u>not</u> IgM like ABO groups)

Figure 15.2 RhD groups and antibodies.

anti-Jkᵃ (Kidd system) and anti-S (part of the MNS blood group system). These antigens are relatively poorly immunogenic. Their potency in stimulating antibody production is 10–1000 times less than that of RhD. Consequently, these antigens need not be routinely assessed prior to transfusion, although more care is required in patients who receive many transfusions (e.g. in transfusion-dependent thalassaemia), as the lifetime likelihood of immunization by these antigens is higher in heavily transfused patients.

Cross-matching and compatibility

The purpose of cross-matching blood before transfusion is to ensure that there is no antibody present in the recipient's plasma that will react with any antigen on the donor's cells. The basic technique for detecting such antibodies relies on their ability to agglutinate red cells that bear the appropriate antigen. If there is agglutination when the donor and recipient samples are mixed, this indicates they are incompatible.

Many red cell antibodies are unable to bring about agglutination on their own and many require additional proteolytic treatment of the red cells or the use of an antiglobulin reagent (see below). The ability of antibodies to agglutinate untreated red cells depends partly on the molecular structure of the antibody. Pentameric IgM antibodies, which readily span adjacent red cells, can bring about agglutination without the addition of any other reagents. By contrast, the smaller IgG antibodies, which are far more common than IgM, do not usually cause agglutination.

Antiglobulin test

The antiglobulin test was first described by Moreschi in 1908, and its relevance to clinical practice was highlighted by Coombs, Mourant and Race in 1945. Its purpose is to detect antibodies to red cell surface constituents, either bound to the red cell surface or free in the serum.

The basic constituent of an antiglobulin serum is anti-human IgG, which is obtained by injecting human IgG into animals and then harvesting the antibodies produced by the animal's immune response. Being bivalent, the antiglobulin is able to bring about agglutination of IgG-coated red cells by linking IgG molecules on one red cell with those on an adjacent red cell, thus holding the cells together as agglutinates.

The antiglobulin test can be used in two ways. First, it can be used to detect antibody already on the patient's cells *in vivo*. Red cells are washed to remove the free IgG in the plasma, which would otherwise react with and neutralize the antiglobulin. After washing, anti-human globin is added and if the red cells are coated with antibody, agglutination takes place. This is the *direct antiglobulin test*, used in the diagnosis of autoimmune haemolytic anaemia and described in Chapter 3. Alternatively, the test can be used to detect the presence of antibody in serum, as in the cross-matching of blood for transfusion. In this case, serum from the patient who requires transfusion is incubated with donor red cells. Any antibody present in the recipient's serum that has specificity for antigens on the donor's cells will interact with those cells. After washing, addition of anti-human globulin will bring about red cell agglutination. This is the *indirect antiglobulin test*.

Procedure for obtaining compatible blood

The ABO and RhD group of the recipient must first be determined by the addition of agglutinating anti-A and anti-B to the red cells. The result is checked by determining whether anti-A or anti-B is present in the recipient's serum; this is done by adding known group A and B cells. The RhD group is also determined using an agglutinating IgM anti-D or by using IgG anti-D combined with the antiglobulin test.

Donor blood of the appropriate ABO and RhD group is then selected. Before this can be transfused, cross-matching must be carried out, partly to ensure that there have been no errors in the determination of the ABO group of the donor and recipient, and partly to ensure that no other antibodies are present in the recipient that react with the donor's red cells. A search is made for both agglutinating and non-agglutinating antibodies, the latter with the antiglobulin test.

The sera of all recipients will also be screened for the presence of antibodies such as anti-K, anti-Fy^a and anti-Jk^a, using a panel of red cells of known phenotype.

If RhD-negative donor blood is not available for RhD-negative recipients, the question arises whether it is safe to give RhD-positive blood. RhD-negative males, especially elderly males, may receive RhD-positive blood provided that care is taken to search for anti-RhD antibodies before any subsequent transfusions of RhD-positive blood are given. However, RhD-positive blood should be avoided for RhD-negative girls or women of child-bearing potential, to avoid stimulating anti-D production with the risk of haemolytic disease of the newborn in subsequent pregnancies.

Haemolytic disease of the fetus and newborn

Haemolytic disease of the fetus and newborn (HDN) is a major example of the clinical significance of blood groups, and arises as a consequence of a pregnant mother having an IgG antibody against a red cell antigen on the red cells of the fetus she is carrying (Figure 15.3). These IgG antibodies may cross the placenta, leading to haemolysis.

Antibodies against RhD (or other antigens) typically develop during pregnancy when a small amount of fetal blood enters the maternal blood circulation. In the UK population, approximately 17% of women are RhD negative. Before the introduction of preventive therapy, a RhD-negative woman, who had two previous pregnancies with RhD-positive babies, would have a 16% chance of having IgG anti-D antibodies. This has dropped to less than 2% following the introduction of preventive treatment.

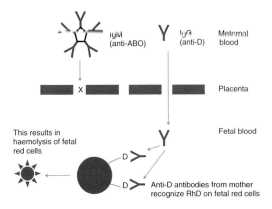

Figure 15.3 Haemolytic disease of the fetus and newborn. IgM antibodies are unable to cross the placenta so do not cause haemolytic disease of the fetus and newborn. IgG antibodies such as those against RhD are able to cross the placenta and if a fetus has red cells expressing RhD, they may be lysed by maternal antibodies.

Table 15.2 The relationship between the number of fetal red cells in the maternal circulation after labour and the subsequent immunization of the mother.

Estimated number of fetal red cells (mL)	Incidence of immunization (%)
0	3.7
0.02	4.5
0.04	10.3
0.06–0.08	14.6
0.1–0.2	18.7
0.22–0.78	21.1
0.8	23.5

Source: From Clarke (1968). Reproduced with permission of John Wiley and Sons.

It is very unusual for the first-born child to be affected with HDN, the incidence being slightly less than 1% of all RhD-negative mothers who have no history of transfusion or abortion. This is because it is uncommon for significant numbers of fetal red cells to cross the placenta sufficiently early in pregnancy to stimulate anti-D production before the child is born (Table 15.2).

By contrast, during a subsequent pregnancy with a RhD-positive fetus, it requires only a few fetal red cells crossing the placenta early in pregnancy to provide a secondary stimulus for anti-D production. This can usually be detected by the 28th week although sometimes may not appear until the last few weeks of pregnancy.

Before the advent of prophylactic therapy, the overwhelming majority of HDN cases were caused by antibodies against RhD, with 6% from other antibodies within the Rh system and only 1% from antibodies in other blood group systems. During the decade 1958–1968, RhD HDN resulted in about 300–400 neonatal deaths each year in the UK, and an approximately equal number were stillborn. During the 1960s, however, prophylactic anti-D immunoglobulin injections were routinely introduced for RhD-negative mothers in the hours immediately following labour, to bind to RhD antigens on fetal red cells entering the mother's circulation during parturition and therefore to prevent active immunization by fetal RhD. Since then, the incidence of HDN has been greatly reduced, and by the year 2000 only about 10–20 fetal deaths occurred annually in the UK as a result of anti-RhD HDN.

Without treatment, the mortality rate of affected infants is about 20%, but antenatal prophylaxis together with the introduction of treatment by exchange transfusion has considerably reduced this. Approximately 60% of affected infants require an exchange transfusion and efficient treatment results in the survival of about 95% of all affected infants.

Clinical features

There is great variation in the severity of the disease in an affected child. In the mildest cases, infants are not anaemic at birth and never become jaundiced. However, the Hb concentration of these infants may fall abnormally rapidly after birth and values as low as 60 g/L may be found up to 30 days later. All neonates with maternal antibodies on their red cells (detected by a positive direct antiglobulin test) should therefore be followed up for a short period after birth.

Moderately severely affected babies may not be anaemic at birth, but the rate of red cell destruction is such that jaundice develops within a few hours. Jaundice is not seen at the time of birth, because prior to this bilirubin is excreted by placental transfer. Within 48–72 hours of birth, the plasma bilirubin may rise to 350–700 µmol/L. The rate of rise of plasma bilirubin is governed partly by the rate of red cell destruction and partly by the degree of maturity of the bilirubin excretory mechanism. As a result of the poor development of the excretory mechanism for bilirubin in many infants, it is quite common for a child with a cord Hb within the normal range to become severely jaundiced. The danger associated with a high bilirubin level is kernicterus resulting from damage to the basal ganglia of the brain, with a clinical picture characterized by spasticity and death from respiratory failure.

In the past, severely affected babies could become so anaemic that cardiac failure with hydrops, or even stillbirth, would ensue. With modern management, such a severe clinical picture is rarely seen.

Management of mother and child

When a pregnant woman attends her first appointment with the antenatal service, blood is taken to check her ABO and RhD status, as well as to examine for any other red cell antibodies that might react with paternally derived antigens. Women who are negative for RhD are at risk of developing anti-RhD antibodies during pregnancy if the fetus carries paternally derived RhD antigens, and these women are therefore considered for routine antenatal anti-D prophylaxis to prevent this. A small amount of fetal DNA circulates in maternal blood during pregnancy. A blood test may be taken from the mother from 16 weeks gestation onwards to check for free fetal DNA. If this shows the fetus is also RhD negative then no prophylaxis is required because there is no risk of haemolytic disease of the fetus. If it shows the fetus is RhD positive then anti-D prophylaxis can be given.

For RhD-negative pregnant women, anti-D will be given as an intramuscular injection at specific times during the pregnancy, with a further dose given within 72 hours of delivery. In addition, any potentially sensitizing event is also treated with additional anti-D administration; such events, when fetal red cells may pass into the maternal circulation, include abdominal trauma, threatened abortion or any spontaneous abortion after 12 weeks. The additional treatment should be tailored to the size of the feto-maternal haemorrhage, which may be estimated using the Kleihauer–Betke technique. This test exploits the differential sensitivity to acid of cells containing fetal haemoglobin and those containing adult globins. Treatment of a blood smear, taken from the mother's blood, with an acid preparation will leach only adult globin from the cells. The cells derived from the fetal circulation can then be counted, and the size of the feto-maternal haemorrhage defined. Appropriate titration of the correct dose of anti-D immunoglobulin can then be performed.

In pregnancies that are likely to be affected, ultrasound examination is useful to detect fetal hydrops, and Doppler ultrasound of the middle cerebral artery can be used to assess fetal anaemia. If anaemia is confirmed by ultrasound-guided fetal blood sampling, intrauterine transfusion may be commenced. As the haemolysis may worsen the longer the pregnancy progresses, induction of labour or Caesarean section may be considered to deliver the baby early.

When anti-D is present in the mother's plasma, cord blood is obtained at delivery and the presence of antibody on the infant's red cells is confirmed by the direct antiglobulin test. Additional essential investigations of the neonate include a full blood count and examination of the blood film for evidence of haemolysis, plus assessment of bilirubin levels.

The usual treatment of HDN involves exchange transfusion for neonates with severe anaemia and/or severe hyperbilirubinaemia (>350 μmol/L) or rapidly increasing hyperbilirubinaemia. For less severe hyperbilirubinaemia, phototherapy can be effective in reducing the bilirubin by inducing photoisomerization to forms more readily excreted without the need for conjugation.

Haemolytic disease from anti-A and anti-B

Haemolytic disease from anti-A or anti-B is almost entirely confined to group A and B infants born to group O mothers; it is mainly group O mothers who have anti-A and anti-B of the IgG class, which can cross the placenta. IgM antibodies cannot cross the placenta. ABO HDN (of all grades of severity) affects about 1 in 150 births. With the advent of successful anti-D prophylaxis, clinically significant disease is now more frequently caused by anti-A or anti-B, by antibodies other than anti-D within the Rh system or, rarely, by the involvement of other blood group systems.

Unlike HDN from anti-D, ABO HDN may be seen in the first pregnancy, because ABO antibodies are naturally present and there is therefore no need for prior sensitization of the mother. ABO HDN is usually very mild; stillbirths do not occur, severe anaemia is uncommon and the neonate rarely requires treatment by exchange transfusion. Phototherapy is usually sufficient to reduce bilirubin levels. A consistent finding is the presence of spherocytes on inspection of cord blood smears. In certain parts of the world, ABO HDN is even more common than in the UK. This may in part result from the high concentrations of IgG anti-A and anti-B in such populations.

Platelets, plasma and granulocytes

As well as red cells, blood from volunteer donors is also used to provide plasma, platelets and granulocytes for transfusion. Each of these has a distinct role in the management of patients with cytopenias and haemostatic defects (Table 15.3).

Fresh frozen plasma (FFP) may be prepared from whole-blood donations or from apheresis collection. Blood is centrifuged to separate out the plasma and cellular phases, and the fresh plasma is frozen for up to 3 years. FFP is typically used to replace coagulation factor deficiencies in cases where multiple factors are lost (e.g. in DIC with haemorrhagic symptoms, or as part of a massive transfusion protocol; see below). A slightly different product, cryoprecipitate, is rich in fibrinogen, and is prepared by thawing frozen plasma in a controlled fashion. As well as fibrinogen, other high molecular weight components are also concentrated in cryoprecipitate, including von Willebrand factor. Cryoprecipitate is often used to replace fibrinogen in major haemorrhage and DIC.

Platelets for transfusion may be derived from whole-blood donations, again by centrifugation. A single adult dose of platelets will require the platelet component of several donors' whole blood.

Platelets may also be collected by apheresis; this more efficient method allows the production of a platelet dose from a single volunteer, thus exposing the recipient to blood products from fewer individual donors. Platelets need to be stored at 22 °C with constant shaking; this has been shown as the best method for balancing function and platelet lifespan, but increases the risk of bacterial contamination. Thus, they have a relatively short shelf-life of 7 days, and supplies need to be carefully managed. Platelets are typically given to thrombocytopenic patients to treat or prevent bleeding. A platelet count of less than 10×10^9/L is often used as a trigger for prophylactic platelet transfusion, although this may be adjusted according to other clinical factors that may increase a patient's risk of bleeding. Higher platelet counts (usually $50-80 \times 10^9$/L) are advised in major bleeding or before major surgery, with platelet counts of 100×10^9/L or more advised before neurosurgery/eye surgery or for intracranial bleeding. For some patients with thrombocytopenia, platelet transfusion is not usually clinically beneficial (e.g. those with immune thrombocytopenia [ITP]) or may even be harmful (e.g. those with thrombotic thrombocytopenic purpura [TTP], see Chapter 13).

Granulocyte transfusions are much more rarely used, and the evidence for their utility is very limited. However, they are sometimes employed in severely neutropenic patients who are critically ill with sepsis,

Table 15.3 **Blood components and indications for use.**

	Red cells	**Plasma**	**Platelets**	**Cryoprecipitate**
Indication	Correction of anaemia	Replacement of coagulation factors	Treatment of some causes of thrombocytopenia	Correction of low fibrinogen levels
Triggers	Major bleeding	Major bleeding	Major bleeding	Major bleeding
	Haemoglobin less than or equal to 70 g/L for inpatients who are not bleeding with no other reversible cause (haemoglobin 80 g/L or less for those with acute coronary syndrome)	Treatment of coagulopathies for bleeding patients or those undergoing invasive procedures	Platelet count <10 × 10⁹/L for prophylaxis Higher targets needed in major bleeding or for invasive procedures (typically 50–100 × 10⁹/L depending on the bleeding risk)	Clauss fibrinogen <1 g/L before invasive procedures; <1.5 g/L for major bleeding; <2 g/L for major obstetric bleeding
	Patients on chronic or outpatient transfusion programmes			

DIC, disseminated intravascular coagulation.

and in whom standard therapies for sepsis have failed to achieve a response. As with platelets, granulocytes may be obtained through centrifugation of whole blood or through apheresis; however, with granulocyte collections, donors must be primed with granulocyte colony-stimulating factor (G-CSF) prior to collection, to ensure that adequate numbers of cells are obtained.

Hazards of blood transfusion: the SHOT Report

As with all medical interventions, the benefits of transfusion must be weighed against the associated risks. A legal framework exists to ensure the best possible safety standards for transfusion, with regulations to monitor all aspects of collection, storage and administration. In the UK, all adverse incidents following blood transfusion are reported to the Serious Hazards of Transfusion (SHOT) Committee. In 2019, SHOT estimated the risk of death due to complications of blood transfusion at 1 in 135 705 transfusions and the risk of major complications at 1 in 17 884 transfusions. Some of the potential complications of blood transfusion are described below, with Figure 15.4 showing their significance in terms of mortality.

Haemolytic reactions from incompatible red cells

Acute haemolytic transfusion reactions are amongst the most clinically significant transfusion reactions, with ABO incompatibility reactions being the most severe. Symptoms may appear within minutes of transfusing ABO-incompatible red cells or plasma, and include restlessness, anxiety, fever, chills, flushing and flank pain. ABO incompatibility reactions may be severe, with circulatory collapse and the development of acute kidney injury.

The immediate management is to stop the transfusion, keeping the bag and giving set so that the transfusion laboratory can check the grouping of the blood component. Circulatory support is essential and, in the context of circulatory collapse, inotropes may be needed. When deaths occur, they are usually the result of either severe DIC or renal failure. The overall mortality following an ABO-incompatible acute haemolytic transfusion reaction is approximately 10%.

ABO-incompatible transfusions should never occur if proper transfusion practice is followed. There are many potential errors that may lead to an ABO-incompatible transfusion, with the most common being administrative (e.g. the wrong patient's details being entered onto a blood tube when a group and save request is sent to the transfusion laboratory). It is critically important to verify the patient's identity at all steps of the transfusion pathway from taking the

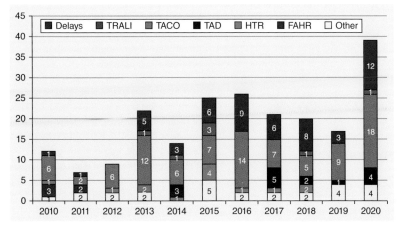

TRALI = transfusion-related acute lung injury; TACO = transfusion-associated circulatory overload; TAD = transfusion-associated dyspnoea; HTR = haemolytic transfusion reaction; FAHR = febrile, allergic and hypotensive reactions

Figure 15.4 Transfusion-related deaths 2010–2020.
Source: S Narayan (Ed) D Poles et al. on behalf of the Serious Hazards of Transfusion (SHOT) Steering Group. The 2020 Annual SHOT Report (2021).

first blood sample for cross-matching through to the final transfusion of blood.

Some hospitals have instituted a barcoding system for blood transfusion, in which the patient's wristband and the sample taken for cross-matching are labelled with matching barcodes at the time of venepuncture. When the blood product for transfusion is chosen in the transfusion laboratory, this too is marked with the same barcode. In order for the transfusion to take place, a barcode scanner must be used to confirm that the correct product is being delivered to the correct patient, with a reduction in the likelihood of the wrong unit being administered. Simple processes such as this can significantly reduce the possibility of transfusing blood matched for another patient.

When haemolytic transfusion reactions are due to IgG (e.g. when RhD-positive donor blood is transfused to a recipient with IgG anti-D antibodies), the haemolytic reaction is extravascular and usually milder. There may be development of a fever, up to an hour after the commencement of transfusion, and biochemical features of haemolysis will be detected (a raised lactate dehydrogenase [LDH] and unconjugated bilirubin, see Chapter 4). This type of incompatibility is almost never followed by renal failure.

Another type of haemolytic complication is the delayed haemolytic transfusion reaction (DTR). This occurs in a recipient who has been previously immunized by transfusion or pregnancy, but in whom the plasma antibody titre has become too weak to be identified. Following the transfusion, a secondary immunological response takes place and the antibody titre rapidly rises, bringing about haemolysis usually around 7–14 days later. Typically, the patient develops anaemia, fever, jaundice and sometimes haemoglobinuria. The temporal dissociation from the transfusion can make the diagnosis difficult. Antibodies to the red cell antigens Kidd (Jk) and the Rh system are the most common cause of these reactions.

Transfusion-transmitted infections

Transfusion-transmitted infections (TTIs) are relatively unusual complications of transfusion because of the adoption of robust safety strategies in transfusion practice.

The majority of TTIs are caused by bacterial contamination of the blood component, which is more common in platelet components because of their storage conditions. Other theoretical TTIs include hepatitis B (HBV), hepatitis C (HCV), hepatitis E, human T-cell leukaemia virus (HTLV) and human immunodeficiency virus (HIV) infection. As would be expected, highly rigorous screening programmes of donor blood are used to ensure that infected components do not enter the blood supply. For hepatitis C, for example, a combination of serological tests and nucleic acid amplification tests to detect viral RNA has reduced the risk of contracting HCV from a transfusion in the UK to an estimated 1 in 28 million. A combination of serological and molecular testing is also employed to screen all samples for HBV, HIV, HTLV and syphilis, among other infections. The estimated chance that a blood unit infected with HIV might enter the UK supply is around 1 in 7 million, and for hepatitis B it is 1 in 1.2 million.

The testing will pick up the majority of cases of potential TTIs. However in the early stages of an infection, these tests may fail to detect evidence of a virus, so the questions asked of the donor before they give blood are essential to reduce the risk of potential transmission.

Another safety procedure that is used for some blood components is the use of pathogen inactivation technology to inactivate viruses, bacteria, fungi and protozoa. The addition of solvent/detergent will inactivate the lipid envelope of viruses such as HBV, HCV, HIV and HTLV, and others such as Epstein–Barr virus (EBV) and cytomegalovirus (CMV). This process is only suitable for non-cellular components (e.g. plasma). Other methods for inactivation of pathogens include the use of photochemical systems such as psoralen-S59 compounds where, after the addition of the psoralen, the blood product is exposed to high-intensity ultraviolet A light. This technology is in use in several countries, where it has the additional advantage of prolonging the shelf-life of some blood products (e.g. platelets).

Bacterial infection may also be detected prior to the administration of the component through the use of technologies such as Bact/ALERT®. This uses a gas-permeable colorimetric sensor and reflected light to measure the production of CO_2 by bacterial metabolism in a blood component product. As CO_2 levels climb, the colour of the Bact/ALERT vial turns yellow, increasing reflectance and allowing detection of the earliest stages of bacterial infection. Frequent monitoring using this system will limit the number of potentially infected units that enter the supply.

Variant Creutzfeldt–Jakob disease

Variant Creutzfeldt–Jakob disease (CJD) is one of a group of transmissible spongiform encephalopathy disorders, and it exists in familial, sporadic and variant types. The pathogenic agent is believed to be a prion protein, which causes disease by affecting the normal conformation of other proteins. There is a long incubation period and so far there is no treatment for the progressive, central nervous system degeneration that this condition produces. Rapidly progressive dementia is followed by early death. Particular concern arose regarding the variant form of CJD during the outbreak of bovine spongiform encephalopathy (BSE) in cattle in the UK in the 1980s. This sparked considerable concern about the possibility of transmission of the responsible prion through the food chain, with the development of the disease after consuming beef from affected cattle. The long incubation period raised the spectre of many potentially infected yet asymptomatic people.

It was also reported that vCJD can be transmitted by blood transfusion. As a precaution, UK blood services exclude any potential blood donors who received blood products from or gave blood to individuals who subsequently developed vCJD, or who have received a blood transfusion since 1980. In addition, all units of blood are leucodepleted to reduce potentially infected white cells from donors transmitting the disease. There is currently no screening test for vCJD.

Cytomegalovirus

Cytomegalovirus is a DNA herpes virus associated with leucocytes, and may be transmitted via respiratory secretions, sexually and during childbirth. The incidence of CMV antibodies varies in different parts of the world, from 30% to 80% or more. As with most herpes viruses, the virus persists latently after infection.

In immunocompetent people, the disease caused by CMV varies from a subclinical infection to the appearance of lymphadenopathy and a mild hepatitis. The main danger of CMV infection is in infants and immunocompromised patients and thus prevention of CMV infection through blood transfusion is targeted to defined patient groups. Premature neonates of low birth weight born to mothers without anti-CMV antibody are especially at risk. Patients receiving bone marrow and solid organ transplants are also at risk (see Chapter 12). Thus CMV antibody-negative blood is generally made available for these patients, although leucodepletion (which is now standard) may offer a similar degree of protection against transfusion-transmitted CMV infection.

Hepatitis E

Transfusion haematologists must remain alert to changes in the frequency of transmission of significant infections, and must assess their potential impact if infection is potentially transmitted via blood component transfusion. Following an increase in the number of cases of hepatitis E infection reported in England, the UK's blood service reviewed its practice on screening for this virus in blood products. Although hepatitis E is typically mild and self-limiting in otherwise well individuals, the virus can be difficult to clear for those patients who are immunocompromised, and chronic hepatitis or cirrhosis may result. The service has offered hepatitis E-negative blood components for transfusion recipients who had undergone allogeneic bone marrow transplantation or solid organ transplants from 2016.

Other infections

Other infections known to be transmitted by transfusion include syphilis and malaria. The prevention of transmission of syphilis is by serological testing of donors. Another factor of importance is the storage of blood at 4 °C, because spirochaetes do not survive for more than a few days under these conditions. With regard to malaria, individuals who have returned from any area where malaria is endemic are not accepted as donors for 6 months. Anyone with a positive malaria antibody test is routinely debarred from donation. Brucellosis, babesiosis, Chagas disease (caused by *Trypanosoma cruzi*), West Nile virus (prevalent in the USA and Canada) and parvovirus B19, which is not inactivated by detergent methods, have also been transmitted by transfusion. COVID-19 has not been found to be transmitted by blood transfusion.

As new diseases emerge from time to time, the risk of TTI always remains. It is therefore important that transfusion is only given when essential for survival or quality of life, so that the benefits clearly outweigh the uncertain risks of TTI.

Transfusion-associated graft-versus-host disease

Transfusion of viable white cells in blood products can in very rare circumstances lead to transfusion-associated graft-versus-host disease (TA-GVHD). This typically fatal disorder is seen in patients with compromised immune function, but may also occur when a patient receives a blood component from a donor who shares an HLA haplotype. Either of these situations means that the transfused lymphocytes are not cleared in the normal way but can engraft and function in the recipient, leading to a clinical picture that usually includes a rash and marrow failure.

The risk of the condition can be eliminated by irradiating cellular blood products (red cells, platelets) before administration. Irradiation is not used for all cellular blood products because it significantly reduces their shelf-life. Patients undergoing bone marrow transplantation, those with Hodgkin lymphoma and patients who have received purine analogue chemotherapy (e.g. fludarabine) are among those who should receive only irradiated blood products to avoid this complication.

Immediate-type hypersensitivity

Hypersensitivity reactions may occur soon after the transfusion of blood or plasma. In mild cases, features may be limited to urticaria, erythema, maculopapular rash or periorbital oedema. In the more severe reactions, hypotension may occur; bronchospasm and laryngeal oedema are rare. In the majority of cases, no cause for the anaphylaxis is found and it is very unlikely to recur with subsequent blood transfusions so no future precautions are necessary. Patients at greater risk of recurrent anaphylaxis from blood transfusions are those with total IgA deficiency and anti-IgA antibodies. For these patients, the risk of anaphylaxis is elevated for future transfusions, which should be with blood components from IgA-deficient donors to minimize the risk of future reactions.

Mild hypersensitivity reactions of any cause probably occur in about 1–3% of transfusions. There is no specific treatment for mild reactions and the historic approach of giving patients antihistamines (with or without steroids) is no longer recommended due to a lack of efficacy. Severe (anaphylactic) reactions are very infrequent and these may require the administration of intramuscular adrenaline.

Transfusion-related acute lung injury

Transfusion-related acute lung injury (TRALI) typically arises after the transfusion of plasma-rich blood components, and is thought to be caused by the interaction of donor anti-human neutrophil antibodies reacting against recipient human neutrophil antigens. Additional 'hits' are thought to be needed in order for the clinical picture to emerge, as TRALI is most often seen in patients already ill with pulmonary pathology.

The symptoms and signs of TRALI typically arise within 6 hours of transfusion, with dyspnoea and hypotension being accompanied by bilateral infiltrates on the chest x-ray. The differential diagnosis of transfusion-associated circulatory overload is best excluded by examining the central venous pressure; while in fluid overload central venous pressure is high, in TRALI it would be expected to be low. Management is supportive, and donors from whom implicated blood products were prepared are excluded from donating further components.

Transfusion-associated circulatory overload

Circulatory overload with consequent cardiac failure can easily be brought about by the too-rapid transfusion of blood components, especially in the elderly and those who have been severely anaemic for some time. This is now the most common cause of death due to transfusions in many counties including the UK, United States and Canada. Blood transfusion places recipients at greater risk of circulatory overload compared to an equivalent volume of other fluid (such as 0.9% sodium chloride). The risk can be reduced by transfusing a single unit of blood at a time (and then reassessing before further transfusions) and giving blood more slowly to those at heightened risk of fluid overload, such as people with heart failure.

The first signs of transfusion-associated circulatory overload are dyspnoea, crepitations at the lung bases and a rise in jugular venous pressure. Stopping the transfusion is the first therapeutic manoeuvre, followed by diuresis (usually with a loop diuretic such as furosemide) if needed.

Iron overload

Transfusion of many units of red cells (typically more than 20) may lead to iron loading, since each red cell transfusion contains 200–250 mg iron, and the human body has no mechanism for excreting this excess iron. Iron may be deposited in the liver, heart and endocrine glands, leading to organ failure. These complications can be prevented by the use of iron chelators to remove iron from the circulation; a similar effect can be achieved with venesection where this is possible.

Febrile non-haemolytic transfusion reactions

Mild rises in temperature (usually less than 1 °C) are common during transfusion. They should trigger more frequent observations during transfusion but should not lead to discontinuation of the transfusion unless other features develop (such as hypotension, tachycardia or signs of haemolysis) that are indicative of a more severe transfusion reaction.

Management of transfusion reactions

For patients who become acutely unwell during a transfusion, the urgent diagnoses to consider are an acute haemolytic transfusion reaction, bacterial contamination of the blood and anaphylaxis.

A potential ABO-incompatible acute transfusion reaction should be considered for any patient with fever, tachycardia hypotension, dyspnoea or chest/abdominal pain. The first action is always to stop the transfusion and clarify that the correct patient's details are on the component being transfused. Any suspicion of ABO incompatibility should lead to the cessation of transfusion, the institution of circulatory support with IV fluids, careful monitoring of pulse, blood pressure and urine output, and supportive management of any developing DIC. The component bag should be returned to the transfusion laboratory with a fresh cross-match sample from the patient; if incompatible cells have been transfused, they may still be detectable in the patient's blood. Samples should also be sent to assess for intravascular haemolysis, including a full blood count, reticulocyte count, bilirubin, serum haptoglobin, lactate dehydrogenase and urine to assess for haemoglobinuria. It is essential that the transfusion laboratory is informed of the potential reaction. This is to assist with the investigation of the potential transfusion reaction and to ensure that other patients are not also at risk if there has been misidentification of samples.

Other haemolytic reactions, although unlikely to be as severe, should be managed in similar fashion. It is important to ensure that the possibility of bacterially contaminated units has been addressed through taking blood cultures. If necessary, broad-spectrum antibiotics may be commenced empirically after cultures have been drawn.

Severe allergic reactions should be treated initially by stopping the transfusion and returning the unit to the laboratory, as above. Intramuscular adrenaline should be considered the first-line treatment for anaphylaxis.

In addition to the reactions described above, acute dyspnoea can occur as a result of circulatory overload (with an elevated venous pressure being a key physical sign) and in TRALI. Diuresis is clearly indicated in the former, while the latter is treated supportively, with ventilatory support where needed.

With mild fevers only, simple interventions may suffice (e.g. giving an antipyretic and slowing the transfusion); similarly, if a mild allergic reaction is evident (e.g. urticaria), chlorpheniramine followed by a slower reinstatement of the transfusion may help.

Delayed transfusion reactions may be harder to diagnose and investigate, because the temporal association with the transfusion is lost. However, it is still important to establish the nature of the reaction so that future transfusions may be managed effectively. Appropriate investigations include a full blood count, direct antiglobulin test, serum bilirubin and assessment of renal function. Treatment is rarely needed, but the expected rise in haemoglobin after transfusion may not be seen.

Massive transfusion

Patients with acute haemorrhage (i.e. loss of red cells and plasma) may require transfusion with large quantities of packed red cells. Massive transfusion has been defined as the replacement of one blood volume over 24 hours, or the replacement of 50% of circulating volume in 3 hours. In such emergencies, it is critical that there is good communication between the clinicians responsible for the patient and the staff of the blood transfusion laboratory; hospitals will have a major haemorrhage policy to facilitate this. In an emergency when a patient's blood group is unknown, group O blood can be administered; however, group-compatible blood can usually be available rapidly after a cross-match sample arrives in the laboratory, obviating the need for ongoing use of 'universal donor' group O RhD-negative blood.

With the transfusion of many units of packed red cells, the patient may become deficient in key plasma components such as clotting factors, and may also become thrombocytopenic (even in the absence of DIC). There is limited evidence to guide transfusion practice in this field, but the administration of one unit of FFP per unit of red cells may be effective in replacing clotting factors. Fibrinogen and platelets should also be replaced, with 2 units of cryoprecipitate and 1 adult dose of platelets per 6–8 units of packed red cells. Wherever possible, this general approach should be personalized by laboratory testing of the full blood count and coagulation profile.

Index

Haematology Lecture Notes, Eleventh Edition. Deborah Hay, Andrew King and Michael Desborough.
© 2023 John Wiley & Sons Ltd. Published 2023 by John Wiley & Sons Ltd.
Companion website: www.wiley.com/go/Hay/Haematology/11e